The Science of Tooth Whitening

The Science of Tooth Whitening:

Bright Smiles, Dark Chemistry

By

Kashaf Raza, Neha Verma,
Dakshita Joy Sinha, Sarita Singh
and Nidhi Sharma

Cambridge Scholars
Publishing

The Science of Tooth Whitening: Bright Smiles, Dark Chemistry

By Kashaf Raza, Neha Verma, Dakshita Joy Sinha, Sarita Singh and Nidhi Sharma

This book first published 2026

Cambridge Scholars Publishing

Lady Stephenson Library, Newcastle upon Tyne, NE6 2PA, UK

British Library Cataloguing in Publication Data
A catalogue record for this book is available from the British Library

ISBN: 978-1-0364-7594-9
ISBN (Ebook): 978-1-0364-7595-6

CONTENTS

CHAPTER 1

INTRODUCTION

DR. NEHA VERMA

Teeth bleaching represents a conservative aesthetic procedure that has gained widespread acceptance in contemporary dentistry for its ability to significantly enhance tooth whiteness. As a relatively non-invasive approach, it offers patients the opportunity to improve the visual appeal of their teeth without the need for extensive restorative procedures. The success of teeth bleaching is highly contingent upon the accurate identification of the underlying aetiology of discolouration, as this directly influences both the selection of the treatment protocol and the expected clinical outcome. In dental practice, tooth discolouration is broadly classified into two main categories: intrinsic and extrinsic, a distinction that is fundamentally rooted in the underlying pathological or environmental factors responsible for the change in tooth colour.

Intrinsic discolouration refers to alterations in the internal structure of the tooth, which render the staining resistant to standard oral hygiene measures and professional cleaning techniques. This type of discolouration often arises from factors that affect the dentin or the enamel-dentin interface, and its management typically necessitates targeted interventions such as internal bleaching. Among the primary etiological contributors to intrinsic discolouration are pulp haemorrhage, necrosis, calcific metamorphosis, and iatrogenic factors associated with previous dental procedures. Pulpal haemorrhage, in particular, is recognized as the predominant cause of discolouration following dental trauma, where haemoglobin breakdown products penetrate the dentin tubules and impart a persistent darkened hue to the affected tooth.

Extrinsic discolouration, on the other hand, is characterized by the deposition of chromogenic agents on the external surfaces of teeth. These agents can include dietary pigments from foods and beverages, tobacco-related staining, and biofilm accumulation. While extrinsic stains are generally amenable to conventional prophylactic cleaning and polishing, persistent or severe cases may require the adjunctive use of bleaching agents for satisfactory aesthetic results.

The natural hue of teeth is a complex interplay of optical properties inherent to both enamel and dentin. Enamel, with its semi-translucent quality, allows light to penetrate and interact with the underlying dentin, which predominantly dictates the tooth's perceived colour. The polychromatic nature of teeth manifests as subtle variations across different anatomical regions, including the incisal, cervical, and gingival areas. Factors influencing these variations include enamel thickness, dentin density, the degree of light reflectance, and the translucency of the enamel layer. In clinical practice, the dentin's optical characteristics are considered the primary determinant of tooth colour in healthy dentition, while enamel primarily modifies the final hue through light scattering and surface reflectivity.

The chemical agents employed for tooth whitening predominantly comprise hydrogen peroxide H_2O_2 and carbamide peroxide, both of which function through oxidative mechanisms that alter the chromogenic molecules within dental tissues. Hydrogen peroxide acts as a potent oxidizing agent capable of penetrating the enamel and dentin, where it initiates the cleavage of large pigmented organic molecules into smaller, less chromatic components. Carbamide peroxide, a urea–hydrogen peroxide complex, decomposes in aqueous environments to release approximately one-third of its hydrogen peroxide content, providing a sustained bleaching effect suitable for night-guard bleaching protocols.

Several clinical techniques are utilized for addressing intrinsic discolouration, particularly in anterior teeth subjected to endodontic treatment. Among these, the walking bleach technique is extensively employed and widely regarded for its efficacy and simplicity. Also referred to as internal or non-vital bleaching, this method involves the placement of a bleaching paste directly into the pulp chamber. Typically, a mixture of sodium perborate with either distilled water or a 3% hydrogen peroxide solution is used. This combination facilitates the gradual release of hydrogen peroxide, which subsequently interacts with the internal chromogens responsible for discolouration. The walking bleach technique is favoured in clinical practice due to its minimal equipment requirements, cost-effectiveness, and ease of application, making it an ideal choice for both practitioners and patients.

Alternative approaches, such as thermocatalytic bleaching, employ external heat sources to accelerate the decomposition of peroxide-based agents, enhancing their oxidative potential. While effective, thermocatalytic techniques may carry a higher risk of adverse effects, such as external cervical resorption, if not applied with precise control and adherence to clinical guidelines. The careful selection of bleaching protocols must therefore balance efficacy with patient safety, highlighting the importance of individualized treatment planning in aesthetic dentistry.

Night-guard bleaching represents another widely used approach for tooth whitening, in which patients utilize custom-fitted trays containing 10% carbamide peroxide for overnight application. The sustained contact of the bleaching agent with the tooth surfaces facilitates gradual oxidative breakdown of chromogens, yielding uniform and aesthetically pleasing results. The patient-centred nature of night-guard bleaching allows for at-home administration under professional supervision, enhancing convenience and compliance. Additionally, the controlled release of hydrogen peroxide during this process minimizes the risk of sensitivity or soft tissue irritation, underscoring its role as a conservative and patient- friendly approach in contemporary aesthetic dentistry.

Despite the widespread popularity and demonstrated efficacy of tooth bleaching procedures, clinicians must remain vigilant regarding potential adverse effects on both hard and soft tissues. Hydrogen peroxide and related agents have been shown to induce protein denaturation and mineral loss within enamel and dentin, which can compromise the structural integrity of teeth over time. Furthermore, prolonged or inappropriate application may irritate gingival tissues, exacerbate existing hypersensitivity, and negatively impact dental biomaterials used in restorative procedures. Therefore, careful assessment of the patient's oral health status, enamel thickness, and history of endodontic treatment is essential prior to initiating bleaching therapy. Protocols should be meticulously tailored to mitigate potential risks while optimizing aesthetic outcomes.

Advancements in dental materials and techniques have expanded the armamentarium available for conservative aesthetic interventions. Contemporary approaches emphasize minimally invasive procedures, integration of evidence-based protocols, and patient-specific customization. The cumulative effect of these innovations enables patients to achieve their desired smile with minimal discomfort, reduced procedural time, and clinically reliable outcomes. Modern bleaching techniques are capable of restoring the natural brightness of teeth, thereby enhancing self-confidence and overall quality of life.

Teeth bleaching represents a pivotal component of aesthetic dentistry, offering a conservative yet effective means of improving the visual appearance of discoloured teeth. A comprehensive understanding of the underlying causes of discolouration, the optical properties of dental tissues, and the chemical mechanisms of bleaching agents is crucial for achieving predictable outcomes. Both internal and external bleaching techniques, including walking bleach and night-guard bleaching, provide valuable clinical options that can be tailored to individual patient needs. While these procedures are generally safe, clinicians must exercise caution to prevent potential adverse effects and ensure long-term oral health. Ultimately, the judicious application of modern bleaching methods allows practitioners to restore natural tooth colour, elevate patient satisfaction, and enhance the overall aesthetics of the smile.

CHAPTER 2

AETIOLOGY OF TOOTH DISCOLOURATION

DR. KASHAF RAZA

Tooth discolouration represents a multifaceted clinical condition of considerable aesthetic and psychosocial significance. In contemporary dentistry, where patient expectations increasingly demand superior aesthetic outcomes, understanding the aetiology and pathogenesis of tooth discolouration has become indispensable. Discolouration may compromise dental appearance by altering the hue, chroma, or translucency of enamel and dentin, thereby negatively impacting the overall harmony of the smile. Moreover, beyond aesthetic implications, certain forms of discolouration may act as clinical indicators of underlying systemic pathology, developmental disturbances, or pulpal and periapical disease processes.

The phenomenon of tooth discolouration may be classified broadly into extrinsic and intrinsic categories based on the origin and location of the discolouring agent. Extrinsic stains are deposited superficially on the enamel surface and are primarily associated with chromogenic dietary substances, tobacco use, or microbial pigments. In contrast, intrinsic discolouration arises from structural or compositional alterations within enamel or dentin, occurring either during odontogenesis pre-eruptive or after eruption post-eruptive, often making clinical management significantly more complex.

The aesthetic management of tooth discolouration requires accurate identification of the causative factors, as therapeutic strategies such as bleaching, laminate veneers, microabrasion, or endodontic intervention vary according to aetiology. As emphasized by Greenwall, precise etiological diagnosis remains the cornerstone of successful treatment planning in cosmetic dentistry. Similarly, endodontic literature by Torabinejad and Walton underscores the importance of differentiating between vital and non-vital discolouration when diagnosing pulpal pathology that manifests clinically as tooth darkening.

This chapter elucidates the etiological spectrum of tooth discolouration, systematically addressing extrinsic causes followed by intrinsic causes, including both pre-eruptive developmental disorders and post-eruptive pathological processes. A comprehensive understanding of the chromogenic mechanisms involved and their clinical presentation is essential in selecting appropriate evidence-based interventions to restore natural tooth aesthetics.

Classification of Tooth Discolouration

Tooth discolouration can be classified based on origin, timing of occurrence, and underlying mechanism as follows:

Table 1: Classification of Tooth Discolouration

Category	Subcategory	Examples
Extrinsic	Surface stains	Dietary stains tea, coffee, tobacco stains
Intrinsic – pre-eruptive	Developmental and systemic	Amelogenesis imperfecta, dentinogenesis imperfecta, fluorosis
Intrinsic – post-eruptive	Local pathological or iatrogenic	Trauma, pulp necrosis, endodontic materials

Extrinsic Discolouration

Extrinsic discolouration refers to staining confined to the external surfaces of teeth or within the acquired pellicle. It results from the deposition of exogenous chromogenic substances that interact with enamel surfaces through physicochemical mechanisms including adsorption, chemical bonding, and precipitation. The acquired pellicle, a glycoprotein-rich film formed from salivary components, serves as a primary substrate facilitating stain adherence. Variations in enamel surface roughness, microcracks, and surface porosity further enhance the retention of extrinsic chromogens. Unlike intrinsic discolouration, extrinsic stains do not reflect alterations within the tooth structure and are generally amenable to mechanical or chemical removal.

Aetiological Factors in Extrinsic Discolouration

Dietary Chromogens Consumption of pigmented foods and beverages, including tea, coffee, red wine, cola, and certain fruits, is a leading cause of extrinsic staining. These substances contain tannins and polyphenolic compounds which possess high enamel affinity, binding to the salivary pellicle and producing yellowish-brown to dark brown stains. The intensity and distribution of staining are influenced by exposure frequency, beverage acidity, enamel microstructure, and oral hygiene habits.

Tobacco Use: Both smoking and smokeless tobacco are potent contributors to extrinsic staining. Tar and oxidized nicotine components deposit on enamel surfaces, generating brown to black discolouration. The stains often localize along cervical margins and interproximal areas where plaque accumulation facilitates chromogen retention. Polycyclic aromatic hydrocarbons in tobacco contribute to deeper pigmentation, which may resist routine prophylaxis.

Poor Oral Hygiene: Inadequate plaque control leads to accumulation of bacterial biofilm which readily absorbs dietary chromogens, resulting in yellowish, brownish, or greenish surface stains. The thickness, maturity, and composition of dental plaque influence both the colour and tenacity of the stain, with older, mineralized plaque often becoming a nidus for persistent discolouration.

Medications and Mouthrinses: Long-term use of chlorhexidine mouthwash, particularly in periodontal therapy, induces brown-black staining through interactions with dietary tannins and denaturation of pellicle proteins. Similarly, cetylpyridinium chloride and stannous fluoride-containing formulations may produce yellow-brown discolouration by chemical deposition on enamel surfaces.

Metallic Compounds: Occupational exposure or medical ingestion of metallic salts can induce distinctive extrinsic stains. Iron supplements typically produce black deposits; copper and nickel salts may generate greenish discolouration; and silver nitrate applications can result in grey-black staining. The severity and localization are influenced by the chemical form, duration of exposure, and enamel surface condition.

Chromogenic Microorganisms: Certain bacteria and fungi contribute to extrinsic staining through production of pigmented metabolites. Gram-positive rods such as Actinomyces spp. can form black line stains along the cervical regions in children. Pigmented fungal species such as Aspergillus also contribute to green or brown discolouration in specific cases.

Clinical Features of Extrinsic Discolouration

Extrinsic stains are generally superficial and may be removed by professional prophylaxis. Their characteristics include:

- Localised or generalised distribution
- Colour variation from yellow to dark brown or black depending on the chromogen source
- Smooth or rough texture, often influenced by calculus accumulation
- Predominant involvement of cervical and interproximal areas
- Non-pathological, although persistent stains may become aesthetically significant

Prolonged presence of extrinsic stains may result in partial penetration into enamel microdefects or exposed dentine, blurring the distinction between extrinsic and intrinsic staining.

Table 2: Common Sources and Clinical Appearance of Extrinsic Tooth Discolouration

Source	Causative Agent	Typical Appearance	Mechanism
Dietary	Tannins, polyphenols	Brown to dark brown	Pellicle binding, adsorption
Tobacco	Tar, nicotine	Brown to black	Surface deposition, oxidation
Poor hygiene	Plaque pigments	Yellow to brown	Biofilm accumulation, chromogen absorption
Medications	Chlorhexidine, CPC	Brown-black	Chemical binding to pellicle, protein denaturation
Metals	Iron, copper, nickel, silver	Black, green, grey	Surface precipitation, ion deposition
Microorganisms	*Actinomyces*, *Aspergillus*	Black, green	Pigment metabolite deposition

Intrinsic Discolouration

Intrinsic discolouration arises due to incorporation of chromogenic substances within the dental hard tissues or as a result of alterations in enamel and dentine composition. Unlike extrinsic staining, intrinsic discolouration is resistant to removal by prophylaxis and often requires more complex aesthetic intervention such as bleaching, microabrasion, or restorative treatment. Intrinsic staining is broadly categorised into pre-eruptive developmental and post-eruptive acquired types.

Pre-eruptive Intrinsic Discolouration

Pre-eruptive intrinsic discolouration develops during odontogenesis and is integrated into the structure of enamel or dentine during mineralisation. These discolourations reflect disturbances in amelogenesis or dentinogenesis caused by genetic defects, metabolic disorders, or systemic insults during tooth development. The severity and clinical presentation depend on the timing, duration, and nature of the etiological factor affecting tooth germ development. Such stains are typically diffuse, bilateral, and symmetrical, and may affect both primary and permanent dentitions.

Aetiological Conditions Associated with Pre-eruptive Discolouration

Deficiency of the enzyme homogentisate-1,2-dioxygenase causes the uncommon metabolic condition alkaptonuria, in which homogentisic acid HGA accumulates throughout the body. Colouration of cartilage, sclera, and skin that is bluish-black in appearance is known as ochronosis, which is caused by the deposition of HGA in connective tissues. In teeth, HGA may become incorporated within the dentinal matrix during development, leading to a brownish or grey-black intrinsic discolouration. Although enamel appears structurally normal, dentine assumes a darker hue, resulting in an overall discoloured appearance.

Amelogenesis Imperfecta AI: comprises a group of hereditary enamel defects transmitted predominantly as an autosomal dominant trait. The condition disrupts enamel matrix formation, mineralisation, or maturation, giving rise to hypoplastic, hypocalcified, or hypomature enamel phenotypes. Clinically, teeth affected by AI exhibit enamel that is thin, rough, and deficient in mineral content, resulting in yellow, brown, or opaque white discolouration. Hypocalcified types present with soft enamel that readily absorbs chromogens, exacerbating discolouration over time. AI is frequently associated with sensitivity, rapid wear, and aesthetic impairment.

Dentinogenesis Imperfecta: A hereditary condition that impacts dentine production is known as dentinogenesis imperfecta DI. Mutations in the DSPP gene are frequently linked to this condition. Obliterated pulp chambers, cervical constriction, and bulbous crowns are seen in teeth. Clinically, affected teeth display a characteristic opalescent sheen with blue-grey or amber-brown discolouration. Enamel may fracture easily due to poor dentino-enamel junction integrity, exposing the darker underlying dentine and worsening the discolouration.

The uncommon genetic illness known as congenital erythropoietic porphyria is brought on by a buildup of porphyrins due to a lack of uroporphyrinogen III synthase. These pigmented molecules become incorporated into dentine during tooth development, producing red-brown discolouration known as erythrodontia. Under ultraviolet light, affected teeth fluoresce bright red due to porphyrin content. The discolouration is permanent and affects both primary and permanent teeth.

Congenital Hyperbilirubinaemia: Raised levels of serum bilirubin during neonatal development, as seen in haemolytic disease of the newborn, Rh incompatibility, or hepatic dysfunction, may lead to bilirubin deposition within developing dentine. The resultant intrinsic staining presents as yellow, yellow-green, or blue-green discolouration termed "bilirubin staining". The severity depends on the timing and duration of hyperbilirubinaemia during dentinogenesis.

Sickle Cell Anaemia, a hereditary haemoglobinopathy, may impair odontogenesis through chronic hypoxia and systemic complications. Affected individuals may develop enamel hypomineralisation and dentinal defects, resulting in yellowish-brown discolouration. Delayed eruption, pulp canal sclerosis, and increased susceptibility to infection may also accompany the intrinsic colour alteration.

Thalassaemia, a genetic defect in haemoglobin synthesis, causes chronic haemolysis and compensatory marrow hyperplasia. Prolonged iron deposition and alterations in dentinal architecture produce blue, green, or brown intrinsic discolouration. Facial bone changes due to marrow hyperplasia may also contribute to malocclusion and altered eruption patterns.

Enamel Hypoplasia results from disruption of ameloblast function during enamel matrix formation due to systemic illnesses, nutritional deficiency, or childhood infections. Hypoplastic enamel is thin, pitted, or grooved, allowing dentine pigmentation to show through. The discolouration may range from white or yellow mottling to brown stains, with severity corresponding to mineralisation disruption.

Dental Fluorosis occurs due to chronic ingestion of fluoride in excess of physiologic levels during enamel formation. Fluoride interferes with ameloblast function, leading to subsurface hypomineralisation. Clinically, mild fluorosis appears as white opacities, whereas moderate to severe forms exhibit brown staining, surface pitting, and enamel porosity. Fluorosed enamel is more porous and susceptible to extrinsic staining.

Pre-eruptive intrinsic discolouration poses significant aesthetic and functional challenges. Management requires early diagnosis and intervention tailored to severity. Conservative approaches include topical remineralisation, microabrasion, bleaching, and resin infiltration, whereas severe cases may necessitate composite or ceramic veneers, crowns, or comprehensive restorative rehabilitation depending on structural integrity.

Post-eruptive Intrinsic Discolouration

Post-eruptive intrinsic discolouration develops after the tooth has erupted into the oral cavity and is commonly associated with pathological changes in the pulp–dentine complex, ageing processes, or iatrogenic factors. Unlike pre-eruptive defects, which are developmental, post-eruptive discolouration reflects acquired changes that alter the structural or biochemical properties of dentine. The underlying mechanisms typically involve the degradation of pulp tissue, haemorrhage by-products, deposition of secondary or tertiary dentine, or penetration of staining substances into dentinal tubules.

Aetiological Factors Associated with Post-eruptive Discolouration

Ageing: Physiological ageing results in gradual deposition of secondary dentine and increased dentinal sclerosis. These processes reduce light transmission through dentine due to progressive mineralisation and tubular occlusion, giving teeth a darker, more yellowish appearance over time. Age-related thinning of enamel further accentuates the chromatic influence of underlying dentine, contributing to generalised discolouration.

Dental Trauma is a significant cause of post-eruptive discolouration and may lead to intrapulpal haemorrhage, pulp canal obliteration, or pulp necrosis. Following traumatic injury, rupture of blood vessels within the pulp causes extravasation of erythrocytes. Breakdown of haemoglobin produces iron sulphide and other chromogenic by-products that diffuse into dentinal tubules, producing intrinsic staining. Initial discolouration may appear pink internal resorption before progressing to grey or brown as haemolytic by-products accumulate.

- Intrapulpal haemorrhage: Following luxation or concussion injuries, rupture of pulp vessels causes extravasation of erythrocytes. Haemoglobin breakdown forms hemosiderin and other pigmented products that infiltrate dentinal tubules, producing pink, brown, or grey teeth.
- Calcific metamorphosis: Trauma may stimulate excessive deposition of tertiary dentine, leading to yellowish discolouration and reduced pulp chamber size.
- Pulp necrosis: Necrotic pulp releases by-products including sulphur-containing compounds that diffuse into dentine, resulting in grey or black discolouration.

Root Resorption: Internal resorption presents clinically as the "pink tooth of Mummery," where granulation tissue within the pulp cavity reflects through the enamel. Progressive resorption can eventually compromise tooth integrity, with the pink hue transitioning to grey or brown as vascularised tissue is replaced.

Pulp Tissue Remnants After Endodontic Therapy: Incomplete removal of pulp tissue during root canal treatment may lead to persistent discolouration. Remaining tissue undergoes degradation, releasing chromogenic substances that penetrate dentinal tubules. Anterior teeth are particularly vulnerable due to aesthetic prominence.

Endodontic Materials: Certain obturation materials and sealers can induce staining. Eugenol-containing sealers, phenolic compounds, and silver points penetrate dentine, producing grey or black discolouration. Mineral trioxide aggregate MTA formulations containing bismuth oxide have also been implicated in coronal staining.

Coronal Filling Materials: Restorative materials contribute to post-eruptive intrinsic discolouration. Amalgam restorations produce grey-blue discolouration via metallic ion migration into dentine. Composites may discolour intrinsically over time due to resin matrix degradation or extrinsic pigment absorption. Glass ionomer cements and zinc oxide–eugenol bases can also alter tooth colour.

Other Local Factor:

- Intrapulpal haemorrhage secondary to caries or pulpitis
- Chronic periapical inflammation altering dentine colour
- Repeated bleaching or acidic insults that may paradoxically alter enamel translucency and expose underlying dentine chromogens.

CHAPTER 3

BLEACHING MATERIALS

DR. DAKSHITA JOY SINHA

Over the past few decades, significant advancements have been made in tooth bleaching materials and techniques. At first, in the 1900s, in-office whitening of non-essential teeth was the main emphasis. Nevertheless, tooth whitening procedures were revolutionized in the late 1990s with the advent of dentist-prescribed, at-home bleaching, often known as tray bleaching. This made teeth whitening accessible for both in-office and at-home treatments, especially for critical teeth.

Today, third-generation home bleaching materials are commonly used:

- First-generation: Liquid formulations with poor tray retention, requiring frequent replenishment.
- Second-generation: More viscous gels, improving retention and adherence.
- Third-generation: Variable concentrations, with additives such as potassium nitrate, fluoride, and amorphous calcium phosphate ACP for enhanced efficacy and reduced sensitivity.

Prerequisites of an Ideal Bleaching Material

The success of tooth bleaching depends not only on the technique employed but also, critically, on the properties of the bleaching material itself. An ideal bleaching agent must combine chemical efficacy with safety, biocompatibility, and patient-centred usability to achieve predictable and satisfactory aesthetic outcomes. Modern research in dental materials has emphasized that bleaching agents are not universally interchangeable; each product must be evaluated for its chemical composition, pH stability, oxidative potential, and interaction with oral tissues to ensure optimal clinical performance.

Several key prerequisites characterize an ideal tooth whitening material, as detailed below.

1. Neutral pH or Non-Acidic Properties: An optimal bleaching agent should maintain a neutral or near- neutral pH to minimize demineralization of enamel and dentin. Acidic formulations can lead to surface etching, increased enamel porosity, and enhanced susceptibility to caries and erosion. Neutral or non-acidic agents reduce the risk of mineral loss and preserve enamel microhardness, ensuring that the aesthetic improvement does not come at the expense of structural integrity. Maintaining a neutral pH also limits the potential for soft tissue irritation, as low pH solutions are more likely to damage gingival and mucosal tissues upon inadvertent contact.

2. Easy and User-Friendly Application: Ease of application is a critical determinant of patient compliance, particularly for at-home bleaching protocols. An ideal whitening material should be formulated in a manner that allows uniform application across tooth surfaces without excessive manipulation. For example, gels with appropriate viscosity prevent leakage onto soft tissues, while pre-filled custom trays or syringe systems facilitate accurate placement. User-friendly application is essential for minimizing errors, reducing the risk of over-application, and ensuring consistent contact between the bleaching agent and the tooth surface. Simplified administration also increases patient confidence and satisfaction, contributing to overall treatment adherence.

3. Effective and Efficient Tooth Lightening: The primary purpose of a bleaching agent is to alter the perceived colour of teeth by oxidizing chromogenic compounds. An effective agent must generate sufficient reactive oxygen species, such as hydroxyl radicals, to break down conjugated double bonds within chromophores, resulting in visible whitening. Efficiency is equally important; agents that achieve significant colour improvement in shorter durations reduce the total treatment period and enhance patient compliance. Rapid efficacy is particularly desirable in cases where immediate aesthetic improvement is clinically or socially advantageous.

4. Short Contact Time with Oral Tissues: An ideal bleaching material should achieve the desired whitening effect with minimal contact time to reduce potential adverse effects on oral tissues. Extended exposure to peroxide can result in transient tooth sensitivity, gingival irritation, or dehydration of enamel. Shorter contact periods that still produce effective bleaching outcomes minimize the risk of these side effects while enhancing patient comfort. In in-office procedures, this feature allows for controlled, safe applications within a single session, whereas at-home systems benefit from formulations that produce gradual but perceptible results over multiple short-duration applications.

5. Adjustable Peroxide Concentration: Patient variability in tooth structure, sensitivity, and stain severity necessitates bleaching materials with adjustable peroxide concentrations. Higher concentrations may be required for severe intrinsic discolouration, while lower concentrations are preferable for patients with sensitive teeth or minor extrinsic stains. Adjustable formulations provide clinicians with the flexibility to tailor treatments to individual patient needs, balancing efficacy with safety. Controlled peroxide concentration also allows clinicians to reduce the likelihood of adverse reactions while achieving optimal aesthetic results.

6. Minimal Material Required for Results: An ideal bleaching agent should be potent enough that only small amounts are necessary to achieve effective tooth lightening. Reduced material usage minimizes costs, prevents wastage, and decreases the risk of excess gel contacting gingival tissues, which can cause irritation or chemical burns. Concentrated, efficacious formulations also simplify application, ensuring that the bleaching effect is localized to the target tooth surfaces without affecting surrounding oral structures.

7. Non-Irritating and Non-Dehydrating to Oral Tissues: Peroxide-based agents have the potential to irritate soft tissues and cause enamel dehydration, resulting in temporary chalky appearance or sensitivity. Optimal bleaching materials are formulated to minimize these effects, incorporating stabilizers, buffering agents, and moisturizers that protect enamel and mucosa during treatment. Non-irritating formulations enhance patient comfort, reduce dropouts, and support sustained

compliance for at- home or repeated bleaching sessions. Maintaining hydration within enamel also preserves its optical properties, allowing for more natural and uniform whitening outcomes.

8. Safety Without Enamel Etching: The preservation of tooth structure is paramount in conservative aesthetic dentistry. Ideal bleaching agents should exert their whitening action without compromising enamel integrity. Excessive oxidation, acidic pH, or prolonged exposure can lead to superficial enamel roughening or microstructural alterations, which may predispose teeth to staining or increased sensitivity. Formulations designed to prevent enamel etching ensure that bleaching remains a minimally invasive procedure, consistent with the principles of conservative dentistry.

9. Quick Attainment of Desired Results Patients: increasingly demand rapid aesthetic improvements. An ideal bleaching material should be capable of producing noticeable results within a reasonable timeframe, whether in-office or at- home. Rapid efficacy enhances patient satisfaction and may reduce the number of required treatment sessions. Nevertheless, the speed of whitening must be balanced with safety considerations to avoid sensitivity or tissue damage. Research into optimized peroxide concentrations, buffering systems, and delivery vehicles has facilitated the development of agents that achieve significant results quickly while maintaining biocompatibility.

10. Customizable by the Dentist for Individual Needs: Finally, an optimal bleaching material should allow customization to accommodate individual patient variables. Factors such as baseline tooth colour, stain type extrinsic versus intrinsic, tooth sensitivity, existing restorations, and dietary habits influence the selection of concentration, application time, and delivery method. Materials that permit such adjustments empower clinicians to design patient-centred protocols, enhancing both the safety and efficacy of the procedure. Customizable agents also facilitate integration with other restorative or aesthetic interventions, such as microabrasion or veneers, allowing for comprehensive, tailored treatment plans.

Factors Influencing Material Selection:

- Cause, depth, and extent of discolouration
- Location of stains
- Patient expectations and preferences
- Cost and availability
- Lifestyle and oral habits
- History of sensitivity or tissue tolerance

Composition of Commercial Bleaching Agents

Bleaching agents are composed of both active and inactive ingredients. Active Ingredients:

- Hydrogen peroxide H_2O_2
- Carbamide peroxide $CH_6N_2O_3$
- Sodium perborate $NaBO_3$ Inactive Ingredients:
- Thickening agents
- Carriers
- Surfactants
- Pigment dispersants
- Preservatives
- Flavouring agents
- Urea
- Desensitizer

Hydrogen peroxide H_2O_2

It is a somewhat viscous, colourless liquid. Its strong oxidative capabilities and ability to permeate the tooth structure have made it a frequently used active component in tooth whitening solutions in dentistry. Its molecular weight is low enough to allow it to diffuse through tooth enamel and dentin, which in turn releases oxygen from dentinal tubules. The oxygen breaks down the double bonds in the chemical structures of chromogenic chemicals, which are molecules that cause tooth discolouration. These compounds can be either organic or inorganic. These compounds' chromophoric properties are diminished by oxidative breaking of these bonds, leading to an apparent whitening effect. Hydrogen peroxide's bleaching capabilities are enhanced by its capacity to reach deep into the tooth matrix, making it an efficient treatment for both intrinsic and external stains.

Properties and Mechanism of Action

Hydrogen peroxide mainly produces hydroxyl radicals $\cdot OH$ and perhydroxyl anions HO_2^- as byproducts of a redox process, which are extremely reactive oxygen species. Tooth discolouration can be efficiently reduced by these species because they can break down big, complicated chemical compounds into smaller, less coloured bits. Concentration, pH, exposure duration, temperature, and the existence of light or chemical activators are some of the variables that affect the bleaching effectiveness of hydrogen peroxide. Whitening speed and depth are affected by these factors because they control free radical release and agent penetration into dentinal tubules.

Activation Methods

The activity of hydrogen peroxide can be enhanced through various activation methods, including heat, light, and chemical agents such as sodium hydroxide. Thermal activation increases the kinetic energy of peroxide molecules, accelerating the breakdown into reactive oxygen species. Light activation, often using LED or plasma arc sources, induces photochemical decomposition of hydrogen peroxide, further increasing the generation of free radicals. Alkaline activation through sodium hydroxide or similar agents elevates the pH, facilitating the formation of perhydroxyl ions, which are more reactive than undissociated hydrogen peroxide. The choice of activation method can influence both the speed and efficacy of the bleaching process, with in-office procedures frequently utilizing combinations of these strategies to achieve rapid aesthetic improvements.

Concentration Ranges and Clinical Applications

Hydrogen peroxide is employed at varying concentrations depending on the treatment setting and desired speed of bleaching. In-office treatments typically utilize higher concentrations, generally between 25% and 3%, allowing rapid tooth whitening within a single session or multiple short sessions. The elevated concentration ensures a high oxidative potential, enabling effective breakdown of both intrinsic and extrinsic stains within a limited timeframe. Due to the caustic nature of high-concentration hydrogen peroxide, in-office applications require professional supervision, careful isolation of gingival tissues, and adherence to safety protocols to prevent chemical burns or soft tissue irritation.

At-home bleaching applications, in contrast, employ lower concentrations of hydrogen peroxide, generally ranging from 3% to 7.5%, with some commercial formulations containing up to 14%. These concentrations are selected to ensure safe daily or overnight use, allowing patients to achieve gradual whitening with minimal risk of tissue irritation. The lower oxidative potential is compensated for by prolonged contact times and repeated applications, facilitating diffusion into dentin while maintaining patient comfort. At-home formulations are often combined with carbamide peroxide, which gradually releases hydrogen peroxide upon dissociation, providing controlled delivery over extended periods.

Handling Considerations

While hydrogen peroxide is an effective bleaching agent, its high-concentration formulations are inherently caustic and require careful handling. Inappropriate contact with soft tissues can result in mucosal irritation, chemical burns, or increased tooth sensitivity. Protective measures, such as rubber dam isolation in in-office procedures and precise tray fabrication for at-home treatments, are critical for minimizing adverse effects. Proper storage in opaque containers is also necessary to prevent decomposition due to light exposure, heat, or contamination, which can reduce the efficacy and stability of the product.

Research Highlights and Clinical Evidence

Hydrogen peroxide's effectiveness, ideal concentration, and application techniques for teeth bleaching have been the subject of several clinical investigations. There was no statistically significant difference in the whitening results between the two procedures tested by De Almeida et al ,2011, who compared a single 45-minute treatment of 35% hydrogen peroxide gel to three 15-minute administrations. The study highlights how hydrogen peroxide may be used at different times to achieve the same cosmetic effects, giving doctors more control over treatment length based on patient needs and tolerance.

Sulieman et al. 2004 further highlighted the influence of concentration on the number of applications required for desired results. Their research indicated that higher concentrations of hydrogen peroxide reduced the total number of sessions needed to achieve satisfactory whitening, demonstrating the dose-dependent nature of bleaching efficacy. This finding is particularly relevant for in-office treatments, where rapid aesthetic improvement is often desired.

Nathoo et al. 2003 investigated the effects of daily use of 25% carbamide peroxide or 8.7% hydrogen peroxide over a two-week period and reported significant tooth whitening. The study confirmed that even relatively low-concentration hydrogen peroxide formulations, when applied consistently, can achieve noticeable aesthetic improvements, supporting the effectiveness of at-home bleaching regimens. This evidence underscores the adaptability of hydrogen peroxide as a bleaching agent across multiple clinical settings.

Safety and Side Effects

Despite its efficacy, hydrogen peroxide use is associated with potential side effects, including transient tooth sensitivity, gingival irritation, and enamel surface alterations. Sensitivity is generally mild and temporary, often resolving within days of treatment cessation or with the use of desensitizing agents. Careful case selection, adherence to recommended concentrations, and appropriate protective measures mitigate these risks. Research has also indicated that the controlled use of hydrogen peroxide, particularly in professionally supervised settings, does not cause permanent damage to enamel or dentin and remains one of the safest and most effective agents for tooth bleaching.

Carbamide Peroxide $CH_6N_2O_3$

Because of its capacity to emit hydrogen peroxide when it comes into contact with water, carbamide peroxide—also called urea hydrogen peroxide—is a white crystalline substance that finds widespread use in tooth whitening. Hydrogen peroxide is slowly released from its molecular structure and then diffuses into dentin and enamel to oxidize chromogenic chemicals that cause tooth discolouration. Carbamide peroxide, which differs from hydrogen peroxide in its controlled release, is a safer and more effective substitute for hydrogen peroxide bleaching systems used in dental offices and at home. Hydrogen peroxide is the principal oxidative agent in the compound's breakdown into ammonia, carbon dioxide, urea, and matrix penetration and pH buffering.

Concentration Ranges and Clinical Formulations

Carbamide peroxide is commercially available in a range of concentrations, including 10% (e.g., Pola Night), 15% (e.g., Illumine), 20% (e.g., Opalescence Night White), and up to 45% (e.g., Opalescence Quick). For most tooth whitening applications, concentrations typically range from 10% to 35%, with higher concentrations reserved for accelerated or intracoronal bleaching procedures. Specifically, a 35% carbamide peroxide solution yields approximately 10% hydrogen peroxide, a 20% solution results in roughly 7% hydrogen peroxide, and a 15% solution produces about 5.4% hydrogen peroxide. The proportional release of hydrogen peroxide is critical in modulating both efficacy and safety, as higher peroxide levels increase oxidative potential but also the risk of adverse effects, such as tooth sensitivity and gingival irritation.

Application Guidelines

For nightguard vital bleaching, lower concentrations of carbamide peroxide, typically 10%, are recommended. Patients are instructed to wear custom-fitted trays containing the bleaching gel for up to hours nightly, usually over a minimum two-week period. This prolonged, low-concentration exposure allows for gradual, controlled whitening while minimizing the risk of soft tissue damage or enamel alterations. Higher concentrations, ranging from

15% to 20%, are recommended for shorter daily applications of 3–4 hours to accelerate the whitening process. Intracoronal bleaching for non-vital teeth often utilizes 35% carbamide peroxide due to its high efficacy and minimal extra- radicular diffusion, providing rapid shade improvement while limiting periapical exposure.

Mechanism of Action and Chemical Behaviour

Hydrogen peroxide, which carbamide peroxide slowly releases, breaks down chromophores in dentin and enamel by producing reactive oxygen species. Carbamide peroxide decomposes more slowly than hydrogen peroxide, especially at ambient and oral temperatures. When applied to teeth, carbamide peroxide continues to bleach for 40 to 90 minutes, in contrast to hydrogen peroxide's near-instantaneous oxygen release. The slow release of peroxide lessens the chances of temporary hypersensitivity or enamel dryness by allowing for longer oxidative activity without overloading the tooth structure. Concentration, application frequency, and contact time with tooth surfaces all impact bleaching effectiveness.

Efficacy and Research Evidence

•Carbamide peroxide's efficacy at different concentrations has been thoroughly investigated in both laboratory and clinical settings. More peroxide radicals are generated at greater concentrations, which speeds up the whitening process, as Bailey and Swift (1992) showed. It is important to carefully determine the concentration depending on each patient's tolerance since the hastened action may worsen side symptoms such as nausea, throat pain, gingival irritation, tooth sensitivity, and bleeding gums.

For nightguard vital bleaching with bespoke trays, the American Dental Association (ADA) has approved a concentration of 10 ± 1% carbamide peroxide as safe and effective. This endorsement underscores the minimal risk to soft tissues and the efficacy of gradual, controlled bleaching. A 10% carbamide peroxide solution decomposes into approximately 3.35% hydrogen peroxide and 6.65% urea, along with ammonia and carbon dioxide, providing a sustained release of the active agent over the treatment period.

Research by Matis et al. (2000) and Leonard et al. (1998) compared 10% carbamide peroxide with higher concentrations (15–16%) and found that although higher concentrations achieved faster initial whitening, lower concentrations ultimately produced comparable aesthetic outcomes when used over longer periods. This highlights the principle that bleaching efficacy can be balanced with patient comfort, particularly in at-home applications where prolonged exposure to lower concentrations minimizes sensitivity.

Three commercially available bleaching chemicals were evaluated in non-vital teeth by Mittal et al. (2015) for their effectiveness whether administered internally or via an internal-external approach. Their results showed that 35% hydrogen peroxide and 35% carbamide peroxide produced the most noticeable shade shift, whereas a lesser concentration of 21% carbamide peroxide produced less noticeable results. This highlights the requirement of using larger concentrations when dealing with extreme intrinsic discoloration.

The effect of carbamide peroxide gel concentrations of 10%,15%, and 20% on the adherence of dentin and enamel to resin composite restorations was studied by Barcellos et al. (2010). Researchers found that when it came to enamel substrate groups, the control grouping had stronger bonds than the 15% and 20% carbamide peroxide groups. Similarly, when it came to dentin substrate groups, the control grouping showed stronger bonds than the 20% carbamide peroxide group. Careful post-bleaching restoration planning is required due to these results, which show that larger concentrations of carbamide peroxide may speed up bleaching but can potentially affect subsequent adhesive bonding.

Safety Considerations

Carbamide peroxide is generally considered safe when used according to manufacturer guidelines. Lower concentrations minimize the risk of adverse effects, such as gingival irritation, mucosal burns, or tooth sensitivity. However, higher concentrations, particularly those used in intracoronal or in-office applications, require professional supervision to ensure patient safety. Protective measures, including custom tray fabrication, gingival barriers, and careful patient monitoring, are essential for preventing soft tissue damage and optimizing outcomes. The gradual decomposition of carbamide peroxide further reduces the potential for abrupt oxidative stress to the tooth structure, maintaining enamel and dentin integrity throughout the treatment period.

Sodium Perborate ($NaBO_3$)

Sodium perborate is a white, odourless, water-soluble powder that has long been employed as a key agent in intracoronal tooth bleaching procedures. Its widespread use in endodontics and aesthetic dentistry arises from its relative stability, controlled release of oxidizing species, and superior safety profile compared to concentrated hydrogen peroxide. Chemically, sodium perborate remains stable under dry conditions; however, upon exposure to water, acid, or elevated temperatures, it decomposes to yield sodium metaborate, hydrogen peroxide, and nascent oxygen, which are the primary agents responsible for its bleaching action. The chemical decomposition can be represented as follows:

$$\text{Sodium perborate} \rightarrow \text{Sodium metaborate} + \text{Hydrogen peroxide} + O_2$$

This reaction illustrates the mechanism by which sodium perborate functions as a bleaching agent. The hydrogen peroxide released penetrates the enamel and dentin, initiating oxidative reactions with chromophoric compounds embedded within the tooth structure. The nascent oxygen also contributes to the breakdown of pigmented molecules, facilitating the whitening of discoloured teeth. The controlled release of these reactive species ensures that bleaching occurs gradually, reducing the risk of tissue irritation or enamel damage compared to the direct application of high-concentration hydrogen peroxide.

Forms and Active Oxygen Content

Sodium perborate is available in multiple forms, each differing in water content and, consequently, the amount of active oxygen released. The primary forms include monohydrate, trihydrate, and tetrahydrate:

- Sodium perborate monohydrate – contains 16% active oxygen, providing the highest oxidizing potential among the three forms.
- Sodium perborate trihydrate – contains approximately 11.8% active oxygen, offering a moderate bleaching effect.
- Sodium perborate tetrahydrate – contains around 10.4% active oxygen and is the mildest in terms of bleaching strength.

The choice of the specific form depends on the desired rate and intensity of whitening, as well as the clinical scenario. Monohydrate is preferred when more rapid bleaching is required, whereas tetrahydrate is suitable for conservative, gradual approaches, particularly in patients with sensitive teeth or high risk of adverse effects. The ability to select the appropriate form allows clinicians to balance efficacy and safety while tailoring treatments to individual patient needs.

Clinical Advantages and Safety Profile

One of the principal advantages of sodium perborate is its controlled, predictable release of oxidizing species, which makes it safer than concentrated hydrogen peroxide, particularly in intracoronal bleaching of non-vital teeth. High concentrations of hydrogen peroxide carry a risk of severe soft tissue irritation, chemical burns, and cervical resorption when used inappropriately. Sodium perborate, by contrast, provides a slower, more controlled generation of peroxide, minimizing the risk of these complications. Its ease of handling, stability in dry form, and ability to produce consistent whitening outcomes have established it as the material of choice for the majority of intracoronal bleaching procedures in contemporary endodontic practice.

Effectiveness of Sodium Perborate Mixtures

There have been a lot of research looking at how sodium perborate and hydrogen peroxide compare in terms of efficacy when combined with water. The results of whitening teeth using a combination of sodium perborate and hydrogen peroxide (3%-30%) or sodium perborate and distilled water were not significantly different, according to studies by Rotstein et al. (1991, 1993) and Weiger et al. (1994). The shade stability of teeth treated with a combination of perborate and water was similar to that of teeth treated with perborate and hydrogen peroxide, suggesting that large concentrations of peroxide are not required for long-term whitening. This finding is significant.

Conversely, Ho et al. (1989) found that, when applied to cases with extremely deep intrinsic discoloration, a solution of 30% hydrogen peroxide and sodium perborate worked better than water alone. According to these results, while water is great for a slow whitening process, adding hydrogen peroxide can make the bleaching process more successful in some clinical situations. It is crucial for clinicians to take into account factors such as the intensity of the discolouration, patient sensitivity, and desired whitening speed when selecting the correct combination.

Comparison with Other Techniques

Freccia et al. (1982) evaluated the thermocatalytic approach, which entails heating the peroxide within the pulp chamber, against the walking bleach technique, which uses a combination of sodium perborate and 30% hydrogen peroxide. Their findings indicated that the walking bleach technique was equally effective in achieving tooth whitening while offering significant advantages in terms of safety and ease of use. Unlike the thermocatalytic method, which carries a higher risk of pulpal and periodontal damage due to heat application, sodium perborate-based walking bleach procedures are minimally invasive and can be safely performed without specialized equipment. This makes the method particularly suitable for clinical practice, where patient comfort and risk minimization are primary considerations.

Mechanism in Clinical Context

The bleaching action of sodium perborate relies on both chemical and physical mechanisms. The slow release of hydrogen peroxide allows diffusion through dentinal tubules, oxidizing the chromogenic compounds responsible for intrinsic discoloration. The nascent oxygen generated contributes to the cleavage of conjugated double bonds within pigmented molecules, converting them into smaller, less coloured compounds. This mechanism is particularly effective for teeth that have undergone pulp necrosis or trauma, where intrinsic staining is prevalent. The controlled nature of the reaction reduces the likelihood of adverse effects such as cervical resorption, which has been associated with aggressive use of concentrated hydrogen peroxide.

Practical Considerations and Recommendations

Before being inserted into the pulp chamber, sodium perborate is usually combined with distilled water or low-concentration hydrogen peroxide in clinical practice. Depending on the degree of discolouration, the patient is summoned back for a follow-up appointment a few days to a few weeks after the mixture is sealed with a temporary repair. If more than one shade is required, the doctor may go over the process again. To avoid irritation, even at lower concentrations, it is important to carefully isolate the gingiva and soft tissues before exposure to peroxide. Thanks to sodium perborate's form and carrier selection versatility, doctors may tailor treatment procedures to each patient's unique needs, all while ensuring the highest level of safety and efficacy.

Inactive Ingredients in Tooth Bleaching Agents

Although the oxidative whitening process is carried out by the active elements in teeth bleaching solutions, which are mostly hydrogen peroxide or carbamide peroxide, the inactive components of these agents have a significant impact on their effectiveness, stability, safety, and patient acceptance. Inactive ingredients, though not directly involved in the chemical oxidation of chromophores, play critical roles in formulation stability, delivery, handling, and patient comfort. Understanding the purpose and function of these components is essential for clinicians who wish to select optimal products and tailor treatments to individual patient needs.

1. Thickening Agents

To alter the product's viscosity, bleaching formulations use thickening agents, also called gelling agents. The gel's flow and retention on the tooth surface are controlled by these substances, which are vital. A sufficient viscosity keeps the bleaching chemical in close proximity to the enamel and dentin, allowing it to penetrate the dentinal tubules more effectively and optimizing its efficiency. Gels can cause soft tissue irritation if they do not thicken properly; improper thickening makes them flow uncontrolled, which in turn causes uneven application, less contact with the tooth surface, and even leaking onto the gingiva. Formulations for teeth whitening often contain thickening agents such as xanthan gum, carbomers, and cellulose derivatives. In addition to stabilizing the gel, these ingredients help distribute the active peroxide evenly throughout the tray or application device.

2. Carriers

Carriers are materials used to deliver the active bleaching agent efficiently to the tooth surface. They influence the release rate of hydrogen peroxide and contribute to the overall stability of the formulation. Carriers may include water, glycerine, propylene glycol, or other biocompatible solvents that ensure the peroxide is dissolved evenly and maintained in a stable form until application. By facilitating uniform dispersion of the active ingredient, carriers enhance both the predictability and consistency of bleaching outcomes. Additionally, carriers can impact patient comfort; for example, glycerine is hygroscopic and can help prevent excessive dehydration of enamel during prolonged contact.

3. Surfactants

Surfactants are included in bleaching formulations to reduce surface tension, improving the spread and wetting of the gel over the tooth surface. Effective wetting ensures that hydrogen peroxide penetrates irregular enamel surfaces and reaches deeper regions of the dentinal tubules where intrinsic stains may be located. Surfactants also contribute to the emulsification of any hydrophobic components within the formulation, promoting chemical stability. Common surfactants in bleaching gels include non-ionic or amphoteric agents that are compatible with oral tissues and minimize irritation. In addition to their physical function, surfactants can facilitate the removal of loosely adhered extrinsic stains by enhancing the mechanical interaction of the gel with the tooth surface.

4. Pigment Dispersants

Pigment dispersants are added to bleaching agents to maintain a homogeneous mixture and prevent aggregation of the peroxide or other formulation components. These dispersants ensure uniform efficacy throughout the application period by preventing localized depletion of active ingredients. Homogeneity is particularly critical for at-home bleaching systems, where extended contact times necessitate consistent chemical activity over hours of application. By maintaining a uniform distribution of peroxide, pigment dispersants contribute indirectly to the clinical predictability and effectiveness of the whitening process.

5. Preservatives

Preservatives are crucial for preventing microbial contamination of bleaching agents, particularly in at-home systems that may be stored for days or weeks. Hydrogen peroxide is inherently unstable and can decompose over time; contamination by bacteria or fungi can accelerate this degradation or introduce additional chemical reactions that compromise efficacy. Preservatives such as sodium benzoate or parabens are often incorporated in small, clinically safe concentrations to inhibit microbial growth while maintaining the stability and shelf life of the product. Effective preservation ensures that the agent remains safe for patient use throughout the intended treatment period.

6. Flavouring Agents

Flavouring agents are primarily incorporated to enhance patient comfort and compliance, especially for at-home bleaching systems worn over extended periods. Bleaching agents can have an inherently unpleasant taste due to their chemical composition. Sweeteners or flavour compounds such as mint, fruit essences, or vanillin improve the organoleptic properties of the gel, making the treatment experience more acceptable. Enhanced taste can increase patient adherence to the recommended wear schedule and reduce the likelihood of premature discontinuation, thereby optimizing clinical outcomes.

7. Urea

Urea is particularly relevant in carbamide peroxide-based formulations, as it is both an inactive and a functional component. Upon dissociation in aqueous media, carbamide peroxide releases hydrogen peroxide and urea. Beyond acting as a byproduct, urea has mild denaturing properties that can facilitate the diffusion of peroxide into enamel and dentin by temporarily altering protein structures within the organic matrix. Additionally, urea can act as a stabilizer within the formulation, maintaining chemical integrity and prolonging shelf life. The presence of urea also contributes to the controlled, sustained release of hydrogen peroxide, which is a desirable feature for overnight or long-duration at-home applications.

8. Desensitizers

Tooth sensitivity is a common side effect of bleaching procedures, particularly in vital teeth. Inactive ingredients often include desensitizing agents to mitigate this adverse effect. Common desensitizers include potassium nitrate, fluoride ions, or compounds that occlude dentinal tubules. Potassium nitrate, for example, reduces nerve excitability, decreasing the perception of pain during or after treatment. Fluoride can promote remineralization of enamel, counteracting minor demineralization that may occur during oxidative bleaching. By integrating desensitizers into the formulation, manufacturers enhance patient comfort, improve adherence to treatment protocols, and reduce dropout rates in at-home bleaching regimens.

Clinical Significance of Inactive Ingredients

The inclusion of inactive ingredients is not merely cosmetic or ancillary; they play an essential role in determining the overall safety, effectiveness, and user experience of bleaching treatments. Each component—from thickening agents to desensitizers—contributes to chemical stability, tissue compatibility, and practical usability. Proper formulation ensures that the active peroxide is delivered efficiently, retained on the tooth surface, and released in a controlled manner, all while minimizing adverse effects. Clinicians must therefore consider the complete formulation, not just the active ingredient, when selecting a bleaching agent for a particular patient.

CHAPTER 4

CHEMISTRY OF TOOTH BLEACHING

DR. SARITA SINGH

The concept of bleaching refers to the chemical degradation of chromophore compounds found in both organic and inorganic groups via a redox reaction. A bleaching agent has the capacity to remove colour from substrates containing double bonds, as well as from aromatic and quinolone structures.

Dental whitening relies on redox processes, which are essentially based on the concepts of oxidation and reduction. One component is oxidized and another is reduced in a redox reaction, a type of chemical reaction in which electrons are moved between different molecular species. Hydrogen peroxide, or H_2O_2, is an effective oxidizing agent when used for teeth whitening. Hydrogen peroxide breaks down when applied to oral tissues, creating free radicals that are reactive. The oxidative breakdown of chromogenic chemicals inside the tooth structure is initiated by these very reactive radicals, which are defined by unpaired electrons. The unpaired electrons of these free radicals are capable of breaking chemical bonds within the pigmented molecules, thereby reducing the intensity of discoloration. In this mechanism, hydrogen peroxide itself undergoes reduction as it donates oxygen atoms or electrons to the target molecules, while the chromophore, or the pigmented component within the tooth, undergoes oxidation. This reciprocal electron exchange is central to the bleaching phenomenon, as it allows for the conversion of visually perceptible stains into smaller, colourless or less chromatic molecules that are no longer able to absorb visible light to the same extent.

The primary active component in most dental bleaching systems is hydrogen peroxide, although carbamide peroxide is frequently employed as an alternative. Carbamide peroxide is a urea–hydrogen peroxide complex that, upon hydrolysis in an aqueous environment, releases hydrogen peroxide along with urea. The decomposition of carbamide peroxide is relatively slower than that of pure hydrogen peroxide, providing a controlled, sustained release of the oxidizing agent. This property makes carbamide peroxide particularly suitable for at-home bleaching protocols, such as night-guard or tray-based bleaching techniques, where prolonged but lower-concentration exposure is desired. The resulting hydrogen peroxide molecules diffuse through enamel and dentin, reaching the internal structures of the tooth where discoloration is localized, particularly in cases of intrinsic staining following trauma, pulpal necrosis, or restorative interventions.

At a molecular level, the bleaching effect occurs through the oxidative modification of chromophores, which are the pigmented molecules responsible for tooth discoloration. Chromophores typically contain conjugated systems of double bonds, which allow electrons to resonate across a series of atoms. The presence of conjugated double bonds is what imparts colour to these molecules, as they absorb specific wavelengths of visible light. It is possible for hydrogen peroxide to oxidize other functional groups linked to the chromophore, break one or more double bonds within the conjugated chain, or cleave the entire conjugated chain into smaller pieces when it reacts with these conjugated systems, all of which can disrupt the electron resonance. Each of these mechanisms results in the conversion of highly pigmented molecules into smaller, colourless, or less chromatically active fragments, thereby restoring the natural whiteness of the tooth. Importantly, the exact pathway by which oxidation occurs is influenced by the chemical structure of the chromophore and the microenvironment within the tooth, highlighting the complex nature of the bleaching process.

The capacity of hydrogen peroxide to oxidize a wide range of organic and inorganic substances underlies its versatility as a bleaching agent. In dental tissues, the target substrates include not only chromogenic molecules formed from haemoglobin breakdown, necrotic pulp tissue, or extrinsic staining but also potentially other organic compounds embedded within the dentinal tubules. The reaction mechanisms of hydrogen peroxide are influenced by multiple factors, including the substrate's chemical nature, the surrounding environment's pH, the temperature, and the presence of catalysts or transition metals. Transition metals, such as iron and copper, are capable of catalysing the decomposition of hydrogen peroxide through Fenton-type reactions, which generate highly reactive hydroxyl radicals. These radicals are among the most potent oxidizing species in biological systems and contribute significantly to the efficacy of the bleaching process. The generation of free radicals through such catalytic pathways underscores the importance of understanding the microenvironment within the tooth and its potential influence on bleaching outcomes.

The bleaching process's efficacy and safety are highly dependent on environmental variables including temperature and pH. Although hydrogen peroxide is more stable in acidic environments, it shows stronger oxidative potential in neutral or alkaline ones. By adjusting the pH of bleaching solutions, one may maximize the release of active oxygen species while reducing their negative impact on dentin and enamel. Hydrogen peroxide's reaction kinetics are also temperature sensitive; higher temperatures hasten its breakdown, boost its free radical release, and quicken its chromophore oxidation rate. But, the danger of side effects, including as pulpal irritation or changes to the enamel surface, might increase with extreme heat. Both professional and do-it-yourself bleaching regimens revolve around this idea of a safe yet effective balance.

Light activation is another factor that has been investigated extensively in modern bleaching techniques. Certain wavelengths of light, particularly within the visible blue or near-ultraviolet spectrum, have been shown to accelerate the decomposition of hydrogen peroxide, increasing the formation of reactive oxygen species. Light-assisted bleaching can therefore enhance the speed of treatment, particularly for in-office procedures, by providing an additional energy source that promotes oxidative reactions. Nonetheless, clinical studies indicate that while light activation can expedite the bleaching process, the long-term effects on tooth structure and pulpal health require careful consideration, especially in cases of high-concentration peroxide application.

The biological implications of the redox reactions involved in tooth bleaching are also of clinical importance. As hydrogen peroxide and its reactive derivatives penetrate enamel and dentin, they can diffuse into the pulp chamber, where they may interact with residual organic tissues. Although low concentrations of peroxide are generally well-tolerated, higher concentrations can induce oxidative stress, leading to temporary sensitivity or inflammatory responses in pulpal tissues. Consequently, clinicians must carefully select bleaching agent concentrations, application durations, and delivery methods to maximize aesthetic outcomes while preserving tooth vitality. Protective strategies, such as the use of barriers over the pulp chamber in non-vital bleaching or precise tray adaptation in night-guard bleaching, are essential for minimizing unwanted tissue exposure.

Furthermore, the structural characteristics of enamel and dentin influence the diffusion and reactivity of hydrogen peroxide. Enamel, with its semi-permeable crystalline structure, allows limited penetration of peroxide molecules, whereas dentin, with its network of tubules filled with fluid and organic components, provides a more direct pathway for reactive species to reach deeper discolorations. The density, diameter, and orientation of dentinal tubules can therefore impact bleaching efficacy, as can the presence of previous restorations, cracks, or calcifications within the tooth. Understanding these structural nuances enables the clinician to predict treatment outcomes and customize protocols for individual patients.

Finally, the oxidative reactions that underpin bleaching are not limited to the chromophores themselves; they can also modify surrounding organic matrices within enamel and dentin. While these modifications are essential for achieving whitening effects, excessive oxidation can lead to alterations in the mineral-organic balance, potentially affecting mechanical properties such as hardness, elasticity, and fracture resistance. Consequently, contemporary research in dental bleaching emphasizes the optimization of peroxide concentrations, exposure times, and adjunctive treatments to enhance bleaching efficacy while preserving the structural integrity of teeth.

Hydrogen Peroxide Bleaching

Hydrogen peroxide functions as an oxidizing agent and possesses the capability to generate free radicals, specifically HO2 and O., both of which exhibit high reactivity, with HO2 being the more potent radical. In its pure aqueous state, hydrogen peroxide displays weak acidity, a characteristic that aids in minimizing its degradation and prolonging its shelf life, while also leading to ionization. This ionization process results in a higher yield of the less reactive free radical O. To enhance the production of perhydroxyl ions (HO2), it is necessary to adjust the pH of hydrogen peroxide to an alkaline range, ideally between 9.5 and 10.8. Under these alkaline conditions, hydrogen peroxide can dissociate ionically, facilitating the formation of the perhydroxyl anion. The perhydroxyl anion can act as the active agent in bleaching applications and can also serve as an electron donor, thereby initiating the generation of additional free radicals. Consequently, the ionization process at these optimal pH levels leads to an increased concentration of perhydroxyl free radicals, resulting in a more pronounced bleaching effect compared to other pH environments. Therefore, hydrogen peroxide demonstrates its highest efficacy within the pH range of 9.5 to 10.8.

The free radical exhibits a high degree of reactivity and possesses significant oxidative capabilities. It has the ability to decompose extensive macromolecular stains into smaller molecular fragments, which are subsequently released to the surface through diffusion. Additionally, it can bind to inorganic structures and the protein matrix (Fasanaro 1992). It is capable of oxidizing tooth discoloration. Various other conditions may also contribute to the generation of free radicals.

Homolytic cleavage refers to the process in which shared bonding electrons are split, resulting in the formation of unshared electrons. This can be represented as follows:

Equation 1

$$HOOH \rightarrow H\bullet + \bullet OOH \text{ or } HO\bullet + \bullet OH.$$

This cleavage mechanism is typically promoted by exposure to light and heat, leading to the generation of free radicals.

In contrast, heterolytic cleavage involves a deprotonation reaction that produces an electron pair, exemplified by the reaction:

Equation 2

HOOH → H+ + •OOH-.

This type of cleavage is favoured under conditions of elevated pH and results in the formation of perhydroxyl anions (Feinman et al. 1991).

Active oxygen species that serve as both anions and free radicals are produced via a third route that arises from a mix of homolytic and heterolytic cleavage. This can be illustrated by the reactions:

Equation 3

HOO• + OH− → O•2− + H2O (in basic conditions) and HOO• → O•2− + H− (in acidic conditions).

Hydrogen peroxide facilitates the conversion of larger molecules into alcohols, ketones, and terminal carboxylic acids.

When decomposition catalysts and enzymes are present, the ionization of hydrogen peroxide can be represented as follows:

Equation 4

2H2O → 2H2O + O2.

Hydrogen peroxide's bleaching power is reduced because this change in reaction dynamics reduces free radical generation. The body's defines against oxygen poisoning relies on certain enzymes that are naturally present in the mouth. As a result, before using any bleaching products, make sure your teeth are completely dry and clean.

Dental Bleaching Mechanism

The process leading to a modified perception of tooth colour can be categorized into three distinct stages:

1. The initial phase involves the penetration of the whitening agent into the tooth's structure.

2. The second phase encompasses the interaction between the whitening agent and the stain molecules.
3. The final phase pertains to the modification of the tooth surface, resulting in altered light reflection properties.

The culmination of these phases results in the observable change in tooth colour following the whitening procedure.

In the context of dental bleaching, hydrogen peroxide permeates the organic matrix of both enamel and dentin. The radicals produced during this process possess unpaired electrons, rendering them highly electrophilic and unstable; consequently, they tend to react with various organic molecules to attain stability, thereby generating additional radicals. These radicals function as potent oxidative agents. The chromophores involved typically consist of conjugated chains characterized by alternating single and double bonds, often incorporating heteroatoms, carbonyl groups, and phenyl rings. By disrupting the electron conjugation within these double bonds, free radicals effectively alter the absorption energy of the molecules.

During the initial stages of bleaching, highly pigmented carbon-ring compounds are cleaved and transformed into lighter-coloured chains. Additionally, existing carbon double-bond compounds, which are typically yellow in hue, are converted into hydroxyl groups (similar to alcohol), which are generally colourless. As these reactions progress, the bleached material continues to exhibit a gradual lightening effect.

Carbamide Peroxide Bleaching

Carbamide peroxide (CH6N2O3) is a white crystalline compound that liberates oxygen upon exposure to water. Research conducted by Moncada et al. indicates that it is available in concentrations ranging from 3% to 20%. In the context of dental bleaching, carbamide peroxide is typically utilized at concentrations between 10% and 15%. A 10% solution of carbamide peroxide decomposes into 3.35% hydrogen peroxide and 6.65% urea. The urea subsequently decomposes into ammonia and carbon dioxide, which raises the pH and enhances the bleaching process. In alkaline conditions, the activation energy required for the generation of free radicals from hydrogen peroxide is reduced, leading to a higher reaction rate and improved efficacy compared to acidic conditions. Additionally, urea serves to extend the shelf life of the formulation and stabilize hydrogen peroxide, allowing it to maintain contact with the tooth surface for an extended duration. Carbamide peroxide formulations typically utilize either a carbopol or glycerine base; the carbopol base is particularly effective in prolonging the release of hydrogen peroxide, thereby enhancing its effectiveness over time.

Movement of Carbamide Peroxide Solution

The carbamide peroxide solution is capable of penetrating the tooth structure and can diffuse laterally or to more remote areas. This property allows for its application on the tooth surface to achieve bleaching effects beneath veneers that are positioned labially. Some patients may experience transient pulpal sensitivity, which could be attributed to the swift movement of urea and oxygen through the dental tissues.

After a duration of 10 minutes of power bleaching, initial lightening is typically observed at the incisal edges and corners. During the initial days of treatment, lower teeth may exhibit a noticeable demarcation line, particularly on the lower canines, leading to patient concerns regarding uneven bleaching. However, it is important to note that this line generally diminishes after a few additional days of treatment. The concentration of the bleaching agent is often expressed in terms of volume rather than percentage of peroxide. Consequently, while these measurements are proportionally related, 27.5% hydrogen peroxide is referred to as 100 volumes, 35% as 130 volumes, and 50% as 200 volumes, which indicates the volume of oxygen released per volume of the specified hydrogen peroxide.

Saturation Point

As the bleaching process advances, it eventually reaches a stage characterized solely by the presence of hydrophilic, colourless structures. This stage is referred to as the saturation point of the material. Following this point, the rate of lightening significantly diminishes, and if the bleaching continues, it can lead to the degradation of the carbon backbones in proteins and other carbon-based substances. Hydroxyl group- containing compounds, which are typically colourless, undergo cleavage, resulting in the fragmentation of the material into smaller components. The loss of enamel accelerates, with the remaining substances rapidly transforming into carbon dioxide and water.

These reactions occur simultaneously, as most materials comprise a mixture of simple and complex chemical constituents. Nevertheless, certain processes are more readily and swiftly executed than others, leading to variations in the reaction rates throughout the bleaching procedure.

Ultimately, the bleaching process culminates in oxidation, resulting in the breakdown and loss of tooth enamel. It is crucial to adhere to the time guidelines provided by manufacturers to prevent reaching the saturation point, where peroxides may become detrimental to dental health, causing tooth brittleness and increased porosity. Optimal bleaching achieves the desired level of whitening, while excessive bleaching can compromise tooth enamel without enhancing whiteness.

CHAPTER 5

DIAGNOSIS AND TREATMENT PLANNING

DR. NIDHI SHARMA

The successful management of discoloured teeth is based on an accurate diagnosis followed by detailed treatment planning. It depends on many other patient's personal factors like:

- The individual patient's desires and expectations about the aesthetic outcome.
- Willingness to spend time in the dental chair and/or to co-operate at home; and
- Acceptance of responsibility to modify behaviour that can affect tooth coloration.

It is crucial to begin with a thorough review of your oral and dental health before whitening your teeth. Using a checklist to collect information ensures that all the relevant details are gathered.

Patient's Checklist

As with any new patient, it is important to obtain or perform the following:

- Consent to undertake an examination.
- Medical history.
- Dental history includes the patient's perspective on dental care, their past experiences, and their expectations.
- A smile analysis is an important part of an extraoral examination that also includes looking for disease and dysfunction in the temporomandibular joint.
- Intra oral examination:
- Soft tissue examination

- Dental examination
- Periodontal examination
- Occlusal examination
- Assessment of the TMJ dysfunction
- Special considerations: vitality tests
- Other information: study models, face bow records, articulated study models.

Smile Analysis and Aesthetics

Bleaching teeth alone may not solve patient's aesthetic requirements. A smile analysis should be conducted prior to bleaching and should be included in the treatment planning stages to determine the smile requirements and the patient's needs. There are many factors to consider when conducting a smile analysis:

- The shape and length of the teeth;
- The lip line
- The occlusal connection between teeth and the smile line.
- There is a sense of artistic harmony since every aspect is significant and because they all work together (Moskowitz and Nayyar 1995).

Patient Evaluation before commencement of bleaching:

1. Visual examination:

The origin, severity, and duration of tooth discolouration can be revealed by a thorough visual inspection.

2. Behavioural history:

Tobacco, coffee, tea, and meals and drinks with intense colours should be asked about by the patient, both in the past and present.

3. Medical history:

Look for underlying medical issues or prescription drugs that may have an effect on tooth colours or be having such an effect. It is necessary to study this history beginning in the prenatal period as many of these issues start at important stages of tooth development. It is important to mention any allergies to plastic, peroxide, or any other bleach components. Particularly for preparations like antihistamines that might lead to dry lips, it is important to include the patient's current drug regimen on the medical history form.

4. Recording of base line data:

Use a high-quality 35-mm camera or an intraoral video camera to record the baseline data. A shade tab that is very similar to the teeth's baseline colour should be included in the photographs. This shade tab should be consistently positioned in each shot, usually with the top left canine teeth as a point of reference. These pictures will serve as a great reminder of the patient's appearance before treatment, which is especially helpful because patients tend to forget how dark or discoloured their teeth were before treatment began and get dissatisfied if they do not see any further changes in shade.

5. General oral examination:

Bleaching should only be considered after a thorough evaluation of the tooth and gum health. A radiographic evaluation, soft tissue examination, and hard tissue examination are all part of a comprehensive oral exam. The teeth need to be assessed for:

- The enamel's thickness
- Existing gingival/cervical recession.
- Prior to bleaching, there was sensitivity
- Even after bleaching, the 'blackish' appearance of transparent teeth remains.
- Spots or opacities of white colour: they will remain and maybe even grow more noticeable as you bleach.
- Bleaching does not remove the banded look that might be caused by tetracycline staining or desiccation on teeth.
- Teeth bleaching is generally a good idea for healthy gums, but it is not a good idea to bleach teeth that have severe gingivitis or other gum disorders.

6. Determining soundness of individual teeth and verifying the vitality of teeth:

A thorough evaluation is necessary to rule out any periapical or other pathological issues, cavities, or damaged restorations, as well as any pulp enlargement that might cause an abnormally high level of sensitivity to the bleaching procedures that are being considered or planned. Inspect the current repairs for damage. If tiny fissures are found, the following procedures are followed in that sequence: sensitivity testing with ice, cold, water, air, and heat. Although microcracks should be thoroughly investigated, they do not automatically rule out bleaching. Bleaching can provide a prismatic look in regions with shallow microcracks, while deep microcracks can enable the solution penetrate the tooth too deeply, causing significant discomfort. The deeper absorption of the bleaching solution causes the region surrounding the micro-cracks to appear lighter.

The vitality of the pulp may be assessed by radiographs and thermal and electric tests. Before whitening, it is important to check the health of each tooth by measuring its vitality.

Important factors to consider when deciding whether or not to bleach a tooth include the kind and degree of stain, the amount of previous restoration, the amount of enamel that is still there, the thickness of the enamel, and other indicators of the tooth's health.

There is less worry about harming nonvital teeth because their pulp does not exist. Prior to whitening, they should undergo endodontic treatment with an effective apical seal. Maintaining the integrity of non-vital teeth is crucial because these teeth can be treated from the pulp chamber or the surface using bleaching chemicals and heat with higher concentrations than vital teeth.

7. Complete prophylaxis

To better evaluate the intrinsic stains and make preparations to remove the discoloration or stain, a thorough prophylaxis using a rubber cup and prophylaxis paste or pumice will erase the extrinsic stains.

Patients With Existing Restorations or Defects in Aesthetic Areas

Patients with matching anterior composite restorations should be warned that bleaching may cause their tooth colour to shift, which might necessitate new composite restorations made of a lighter shade composite. Tooth bleaching causes teeth to become exceptionally brilliant shortly after the operation, thus it is best to wait around two weeks before choosing a final shade for new restorations to finish before scheduling the appointment.

Bleaching helps fix teeth with cavities or restorations that are not up to par. Whitening will halt the lesion's development thanks to the cariostatic activity of the substance. Both the physical debridement's antibacterial effects and the direct chemical effect of hydrogen peroxide on tooth enamel might make this a reality. Additionally, it is believed that this effect is caused by the fact that whitening kits typically contain fluoride, potassium nitrate, and urea, which raise the pH of the mouth above the crucial threshold for demineralization, hence reducing the susceptibility to caries in enamel and dentin.

Special Considerations for Bleaching in Older Patients

Bleaching may be a beautiful and effective way to get rid of age spots. Teeth that have become discoloured with age typically show the most noticeable improvement after bleaching. Since it is feasible to utilize a greater bleaching temperature on older patients due to the pulp shrinkage, bleaching can be a very beneficial therapy for these individuals.

Special Considerations for Bleaching in Younger Patients

Bleaching is safe for patients of any age; however younger patients require extra caution to prevent pulpal hyperaemia. Using less intense in-office sessions or heat-free matrix bleaching are two ways to reduce or eliminate the need for heat.

Shade Assessment and Selection

Choosing the right shade of teeth to bleach may be done in a variety of ways. The pre-operative shade is often determined using proprietary shade parameters. Both the dentist and the patient can benefit from the bleaching kit is individualized shade guide. The problem is that these instructions might not be able to pick up on subtle variations in shade. Arranging the shade tabs according to value rather than hue makes it easier to choose the proper shade before, during, and after bleaching. When evaluating subtle colour shifts following a few days of bleaching, this works well. Factors that determine shade value are:

1. The amount of natural light in the area where the shade is recorded.
2. The hue of the tooth colour (yellow or blue range)
3. The value of the colour, i.e. the lightness and brightness
4. Chroma: the strength or weakness of the colour.

Colour and saturation have no bearing on value. Among the three aspects of colour, it is crucial when it comes to dental shade matching. It is recommended to choose the value first, and then the colour. Looking at the middle or cervical thirds will reveal the fundamental hue the finest. Even in the same tooth, chroma differences can be seen. It is common for the cervical third to have a more intense hue and greater chroma than the middle third. The value of the incisal third is often lower than that of the middle and cervical thirds.66 In order to assist dentists in choosing hues, there have been significant technological advancements. New is the 3D Master Shade System, which is one invention. It is necessary to determine if the discoloration or change in hue can be remedied once the shade has been chosen. According to a rule of thumb that Haywood brought up, teeth may typically be lightened if the shade of the sclera (the white of the eye) is lighter than the original tooth shade. It will be more challenging to achieve good tooth whitening if the tooth colour is lighter than the sclera.

Treatment Planning Discussion and Informed Consent

Having a conversation with the patient about treatment plans is crucial prior to commencing any dental procedure. It is possible to go over the patient's current medical status with them during this consultation. The treatment can be explained and discussed, as well as treatment sequencing

and any further treatment that may be required. The patient should be informed about all related and further procedures, since tooth whitening might not be enough to meet their cosmetic needs. Having the patient sign an informed consent form is a good idea. The pros and cons of whitening and other treatments, as well as their alternatives, should be thoroughly examined. Make note of any negative effects, both anticipated and otherwise.

CHAPTER 6

FACTORS INFLUENCING TOOTH BLEACHING

DR. KASHAF RAZA

There are a number of methods and approaches that have been introduced for bleaching of both vital and non-vital tooth. Various factors are involved in governing such an efficient bleaching. These are tooth related factors and material related factors:

Tooth related factors:

- Type of stain
- Presence of plaque/calculus
- Age
- Gender
- Tooth substrate

Material related factors:

- Type of bleach
- Concentration of peroxide
- Shelf life
- Ph
- Temperature
- Time
- sealed environment
- additives

Type of Stain

The classification of tooth discoloration into extrinsic and intrinsic types plays a pivotal role in determining the prognosis and effectiveness of tooth bleaching procedures. Understanding the origin and depth of the stain is essential for predicting treatment outcomes, selecting the most appropriate bleaching technique, and setting realistic patient expectations. Extrinsic stains are superficial deposits on the enamel surface, commonly resulting from the accumulation of chromogenic substances present in foods, beverages, or tobacco products. These stains are typically associated with lifestyle and dietary habits, such as frequent consumption of coffee, tea, red wine, or exposure to smoking. Because extrinsic stains are located on the outermost layers of enamel, they are generally more amenable to removal through professional prophylactic procedures, including scaling, polishing, and application of mild abrasive agents. Regular oral hygiene practices can also prevent the recurrence of these stains, and in most cases, extrinsic discoloration does not require the application of potent bleaching agents to achieve satisfactory aesthetic results.

On the other hand, intrinsic stains start from the enamel or dentin inside the tooth. Tooth discolorations can occur as a result of trauma, pulpal disease, developmental abnormalities, or exposure to certain systemic or local medications while the tooth is still developing. Some common causes include pulpal haemorrhage and hemosiderin deposition caused by dental trauma, pulp necrosis, or exposure to tetracycline during tooth formation. Tooth stains that are intrinsic are not easily removed by surface cleaning methods; instead, they need bleaching solutions that can penetrate the dentinal tubules and enamel to reach the chromogenic molecules that produce the discoloration and oxidize them. It is essential to carefully choose cases in order to optimize outcomes when using non-vital bleaching techniques, such as intracoronal or walking bleach treatments, on these types of instances.

The prognosis of bleaching is influenced not only by the location of the stain but also by its aetiology and severity. Teeth that are affected primarily by internal factors, such as trauma or pulpal necrosis, often respond well to bleaching, particularly when the discoloration is moderate. Conversely, teeth with a combination of intrinsic and extrinsic staining present a more complex challenge. The presence of surface deposits overlying deeper intrinsic chromophores can impede the penetration of the bleaching agent, thereby reduce treatment efficacy and require a combined approach that includes prophylactic cleaning prior to bleaching.

Additionally, discolorations resulting from medicaments, restorations, or severe structural compromise may be resistant or even refractory to bleaching. For instance, stains associated with amalgam restorations, resin composites, or tetracycline incorporation are chemically stable and cannot be effectively oxidized by conventional peroxide-based agents. Similarly, teeth with severe discoloration often demonstrate less favourable outcomes compared to those with mild or moderate staining. Evidence from clinical studies suggests that initial tooth colour is a strong predictor of bleaching success; lighter teeth tend to whiten more readily than darker teeth. Among intrinsic stains, yellow discolorations are considered the most responsive to bleaching interventions, followed in decreasing order of responsiveness by light grey, light brown, dark yellow, dark brown, grey, and black.

Overall, the type, depth, and severity of staining are critical determinants in the selection of bleaching protocols and the expected aesthetic outcome. Accurate assessment of these factors enables clinicians to tailor treatment strategies, choose between in-office or at-home modalities, and counsel patients regarding the likelihood of achieving their desired tooth colour, thereby enhancing both clinical success and patient satisfaction.

Presence of Plaque/ Calculus

The debris on the surface minimizes the contact of the bleaching agent with the tooth surface. The presence of pellicle and plaque on the tooth surface has the theoretical potential to reduce the activity of peroxide by acting as a substrate for peroxide bleaching and/or degrading peroxide. Complete prophylaxis and polishing should be performed in order to eliminate all superficial debris. A clinical study by Wattanapayungkul et al. (2003) has shown that the rate of peroxide degradation did not increase with the presence of pellicle on tooth surfaces in vivo over 1 h indicating that pellicle does not have a significant effect on the stability of peroxide. In addition, another study by Gerlach et al (2002) compared the effect of immediate prebrushing with a toothpaste versus no prebrushing prior to tooth bleaching with 6.5% hydrogen peroxide over a 14-day period, suggested that toothbrushing immediately before bleaching has only a modest positive impact on overall efficacy.

Age

Aging is a common cause for discoloration. The following factors are encountered with increasing age:

- Enamel changes. There may be both thinning and texture changes.
- Dentin deposition. Secondary and tertiary dentin deposition, pulp stones, and dentin aging all cause the tooth to appear darker.
- Salivary changes. Salivary content and composition may change with advancing age.

Teenagers are a great candidate for this procedure since they are just starting to pay attention to their physical attributes, particularly their teeth.9 Assuming there is enough enamel to whiten, whitening treatments often work well on teeth in this age range. Enamel permeability declines with age, and secondary and tertiary dentin are put down throughout the years, thus whitening will take longer in older people.

When it comes to original tooth colour, younger individuals with more yellowish teeth show the most significant mean colour shift after bleaching, whereas older patients with less yellowish teeth show the least. Changes on both the surface and the subsurface of the tooth cause it to change colour. The degree to which symptoms appear is correlated with the tooth's structure, namely its structural hardness. In a study by Camps et al. (2007), they tested the rate of hydrogen peroxide diffusion through human dentin in two age groups: those under 20 and those in the 40–60 age bracket. A hole was made at the CEJ when the teeth underwent endodontic treatment. Hydrogen peroxide gel (20%) was used to fill the access cavities. At 1,24,48, and 120 hours, the diffusing hydrogen peroxide quantity was measured. When compared to older teeth, younger teeth had a greater diffusive flow and maximum diffusion.

Gender

Patient perception of dental aesthetics is influenced by several psychosocial factors, among which gender plays a notable role. Research has consistently demonstrated that dissatisfaction with tooth colour is significantly more prevalent among female patients compared to their male counterparts. Several interrelated factors may contribute to this difference, including societal expectations, cultural norms, and personal attitudes toward physical appearance. In many societies, women are socialized to place a higher emphasis on cosmetic and aesthetic attributes, including the appearance of their smile. Consequently, females tend to be more attentive to subtle variations in tooth colour and are more likely to perceive minor discolorations as aesthetically undesirable.

Additionally, female patients often exhibit a greater degree of critical self-assessment regarding their dental appearance. Studies have shown that women are more likely than men to scrutinize their teeth, noticing irregularities in colour, alignment, or surface texture that might go unnoticed by male patients. This heightened awareness may contribute to a stronger desire for cosmetic dental treatments, including tooth whitening, veneers, or other aesthetic interventions. Psychological factors, such as self-esteem and social confidence, further amplify the impact of tooth discoloration on female patients, making even mild staining a source of dissatisfaction or self-consciousness.

In contrast, male patients, although increasingly concerned with their appearance in contemporary society, tend to prioritize functional aspects of dentition over purely cosmetic factors. Men may be less influenced by societal beauty standards concerning smile aesthetics and are generally less critical in evaluating subtle variations in tooth colour. As a result, the demand for elective cosmetic procedures, such as bleaching, is historically higher among female patients.

Understanding the influence of gender on perceptions of tooth colour is essential for dental practitioners when planning treatment. It allows clinicians to anticipate patient expectations, tailor communication regarding achievable results, and provide personalized treatment plans. Recognizing that female patients are often more motivated by cosmetic outcomes can guide clinicians in selecting appropriate bleaching protocols, counselling on realistic expectations, and achieving higher patient satisfaction.

Tooth Substrate

The tooth's enamel, dentin, and cementum are its three hard tissues. Different types of inorganic and organic compounds, as well as distinct structural features, are present in these tissues, and these features change with time and in response to both internal and external factors.

Kugel et al. (2007) The researchers in this study looked at the enamel and dentin colour changes independently and then connected those variations to the tooth's total colour shift. They came to the conclusion that the tooth's overall colour shift was due to enamel's colour change and not dentin's colour change. In contrast to this study's findings, McCaslin et al. (1999) shown that bleaching can be applied to dentin as well. What is more, the alterations happened uniformly across the dentin, suggesting that carbamide peroxide may readily permeate the tooth.

Type of Bleach

Hydrogen peroxide and carbamide peroxide have been the subjects of most teeth whitening investigations. When exposed to water, the latter substance decomposes into its component parts, which are urea and hydrogen peroxide, as it is an adduct of the two. A maximum of 3.6% hydrogen peroxide may be obtained from 10% carbamide peroxide gel. Whether studied in vitro or in vivo, the efficacy of hydrogen peroxide-containing goods is roughly comparable to that of carbamide peroxide-containing products with the same or a similar amount of hydrogen peroxide and administered in the same format and formulations.

In a clinical study by Nathoo et al. (2003), There were no significant differences between the products, however after two weeks of usage, both the 25% carbamide peroxide gel and the 8.7% hydrogen peroxide gel significantly lightened the tooth shade compared to baseline. The effectiveness and safety of four gels with different concentrations (10% and 15% carbamide peroxide and 7.5% and 9.5% hydrogen peroxide) used for vital bleaching at home were examined by Alonso de la Peña V et al (2014). The researchers discovered that the products did not differ in the degree of whitening.

Another study by Peixoto AC et al (2018) found that 37% carbamide peroxide (CP) was more effective than 35% hydrogen peroxide in whitening teeth and caused less sensitivity. They discovered that while 37% CP reduced tooth sensitivity, it diminished the efficacy of tooth whitening.

A study by Cullen et al (1993) noted that bleaching solutions containing 30% hydrogen peroxide reduced the tensile strength of composite resins, but 10% carbamide peroxide treated composites did not exhibit a discernible decline in tensile strength.

Lim MY et al (2004) For the purpose of intracoronal bleaching of discoloured teeth that have had root fillings, the researchers in this study tested three different bleaching solutions: 35% carbamide peroxide, 35% hydrogen peroxide, and sodium perborate. Thirty-five per cent carbamide peroxide and 35% hydrogen peroxide were equally effective for intracoronal bleaching, and significantly better than sodium perborate after 7 days. There were no discernible variations among the categories following the fourteen-day mark. The effectiveness of sodium perborate/37% carbamide peroxide paste and standard sodium perborate/distilled water for intracoronal bleaching was also examined in another study by de Souza-Zaroni WC et al (2009)80. For intracoronal bleaching, the combination of sodium perborate and 37% carbamide peroxide is just as effective as the sodium perborate and distilled water combination.

Concentration of Peroxide

Increasing the concentration of peroxide amplifies the bleaching action. A more caustic form of hydrogen peroxide, 35%, is used for office bleaching. Fifteen percent and 20% solutions of carbamide peroxide are available for dentist-supervised home whitening procedures. However, the American Dental Association (ADA) only accepted the 10 ± 1% carbamide peroxide concentration, guaranteeing its safety and effectiveness for at-home teeth whitening.

However, it was found that higher concentrations of bleaching agents require lesser no. of applications for the efficient bleaching. Sulieman et al. (2004) studied the effectiveness of tooth whitening gels containing 5-35%

hydrogen peroxide in vitro and discovered that a reduced number of gel applications was needed to achieve uniform bleaching at higher concentrations. In a similar vein, Leonard et al. (1998) examined the effectiveness of several concentrations of carbamide peroxide gels for teeth whitening in vitro and discovered that the whitening process started off quicker with the 10% and 16% concentrations than with the 5% concentration. With an increase in treatment duration, however, the 5% concentration began to show effectiveness comparable to that of the higher doses. In a clinical study using custom made bleaching trays, Kihn et al. (2004) showed that a 15% carbamide peroxide gel gave significantly more tooth whitening than a 10% carbamide gel after 2 weeks use.

Shelf Life

Carbamide peroxide is more stable than hydrogen peroxide & has a shelf life of 1-2 years, while hydrogen peroxide has a shelf life of just a few weeks.

Temperature

When bleaching in the office, this is crucial. The production of oxygen free radicals is accelerated as the temperature rises. A rise of 10 degrees Celsius quadruples the response. Lights with a wide spectrum of wavelengths and intensities, such as halogen curing lights, plasma arc lamps, lasers, and light-emitting diodes, can activate peroxide, speeding up the bleaching process's chemical redox reaction. Also, it is been suggested that the light source might really power up the tooth stain, which would speed up the whitening process overall. To facilitate the passage of energy from the light source to the peroxide gel, several products used in light activated bleaching include coloured ingredients like carotene and manganese sulphate. But, irreparable pulpal damage results from a temperature rise to an unpleasant level, which in turn produces tooth sensitivity and irritation. The patient should be able to notify the dentist in the event that the bleaching gel seeps through the barriers and causes a scorching or painful feeling, hence local anaesthesia should not be given during the procedure as gel seeps through the barriers to cause a burning sensation or pain.

pH

The pH of bleaching solutions can range from 3.67 to 11.13. The pH of the bleaching chemical is said to be increasingly acidic as the peroxide concentration increases. Both the urea concentration and the amount of time it is applied determine its impact on the pH. Whitening kits typically include urea, which both increases the solution's pH and stabilizes the hydrogen peroxide.

Hydrogen peroxide is active in alkaline nature of pH. Thus, the optimum pH ranges from 9.5 to 10.8 for hydrogen peroxide. Hughes JA et al (2000) examined the impact of pH on enamel and shown that deterioration of enamel occurs at low pH and high acid concentration. Enamel loss can be reduced by half by adding a little calcium to an acidic solution.

Negative side effects may occur if the teeth and oral tissues are exposed to a low or high pH for a long time. Demineralization of enamel is anticipated to take place when the pH drops below the crucial point of 5.2. Nevertheless, the natural pellicle that forms in living organisms and the quantity of mineral ions in saliva should prevent demineralization of enamel.85 In a study by Sa Y et al (2013),

they concluded that In-office bleaching agents with low pH values could induce enamel morphology alterations under in vitro conditions But, the presence of natural human saliva could eliminate the demineralization effect caused by low pH.

Time

The longer you expose yourself to the bleach, the stronger its impact will be. The higher the duration of exposure, the more pronounced the colour shift. Tooth sensitivity, though, develops with extended contact.

A study by Kihn et al (2002) assessed the effect of varying bleaching durations on tooth colour alteration. When evaluating eight different in-office bleaching products (15~35%), another investigation by Matis et al. (2007) found that contact duration (15~60min) was more relevant than concentration.

Shorter the time the tooth has been discoloured, the more successful the bleaching is. In a study by Brown et al (1965) who shown that after bleaching, 87.5% of teeth discoloured for one year or less, 71% for one to five years, and 66.6% for five years or more restored their natural colour.

Sealed Environment

Placing the hydrogen peroxide into a sealed environment has been shown to increase its bleaching efficiency. A new power whitening approach, the "Sealed Bleaching Technique" (developed by Kwon in 2007), uses a linear low-density polyethylene (LLDPE) wrap to keep the active ingredients in the gel from drying up and evaporating. Instead of evaporating into thin air, the activated whitening ingredient in sealed bleaching stays concentrated on the tooth surface and is driven into the tooth itself. This is achieved by creating a sealed environment. This method makes the whitening process safer while simultaneously increasing its effectiveness. The whitening agent cannot evaporate into the air or be accidentally exposed to airborne particles if the container is sealed. The activated whitening substance is employed more efficiently, allowing for lesser concentrations to be used. Additionally, there is no need for replenishment, making the operation easy and cost-effective.

Lee et al. (2010) showed in a clinical study of ten patients using a split arch design that a greater shade difference was observed after whitening in the sealed bleaching group compared to the conventional bleaching group.

Additives

To change the product's handling properties or patient acceptance, many peroxides contain additions. Chemicals like glycerine, carbapol, glycol, etc. are added to bleaching agents to make them thicker. However, these additives change the pH of the agent, which in turn influences how effective the bleaching substance is.

The glycerine basis in carbamide peroxide makes the solution more viscous and easier to work with. But it might cause the tooth to become dry. Some people have a painful throat as a side effect of using these agents. This might be because of the dehydrating impact or because they swallowed the glycerine in the solution.

The whitener's viscosity is increased by carbopol as well. Because Carbopol is thixotropic, it helps the slow-releasing gel stay put in the tray for longer. You just need about 29 millilitres (mL) of whitening solution per arch for the whole procedure. Saliva is unable to hydrolyse the hydrogen peroxide due to its increased viscosity, which may lead to more potent outcomes. Carbamide peroxide needs time to diffuse into the tooth, which is provided by the viscosity, which also increases adhesion.

The field of aesthetic dentistry stands to gain greatly from the ongoing interest in tooth whitening among clinical researchers. This interest will lead to a deeper mechanistic understanding of the factors controlling the whitening process, which in turn will improve tooth whitening products and procedures. Patients will be more likely to comply and be satisfied with the results of the whitening process as a result of this.

CHAPTER 7

CLASSIFICATIONS OF BLEACHING TECHNIQUES

DR. NIDHI SHARMA

Depending upon the vitality of the tooth, bleaching protocol can be categorized as:

A. Extra coronal bleaching (vital tooth bleaching)
- In-office vital bleaching technique
- At-home vital bleaching technique
- Over the counter bleaching technique

B. Intracoronal bleaching (bleaching of endodontically treated tooth/nonvital bleaching)
- Walking bleach technique
- Thermocatalytic bleaching technique
- In-office bleaching technique
- Inside/Outside bleaching

CHAPTER 8

VITAL TOOTH BLEACHING

DR. KASHAF RAZA

The usage of vital teeth bleaching to cure tooth discoloration is on the rise. It is an affordable, non-invasive way to whiten teeth without causing any damage. The most typical ingredients for effective teeth bleaching are hydrogen peroxide and peroxide-realizing agents like carbamide peroxide.

There are various indications and contraindications of vital tooth bleaching.

Indications

1. Mild to generalized staining
2. 'Age yellowing' discolouration
3. Mild tetracycline staining
4. Very mild fluorosis (brown or white)
5. Acquired superficial staining
6. Stains from tobacco smoking
7. Absorptive and penetration stains (tea and coffee)
8. Colour change related to pulpal trauma or necrosis
9. Young patients with an inherited yellow or grey hue to the teeth.

Contraindications

1. Severe tetracycline staining
2. Severe pitting hypoplasia
3. Severe fluorosis stain
4. Teeth that react very strongly to changes in temperature, pressure, and flavour

5. Discoloration in adolescents with big pulps: Adverse effects are more likely to occur in younger patients with weaker enamel and bigger pulp chambers.
6. For individuals who would prefer not to or are unable to bear the additional expense of replacing existing crowns or restorations after bleaching, teeth with poor existing restorations may be a contraindication. Tooth discoloration might also result from a repair that is leaking.
7. Attrition, abrasion, and erosion can cause tooth surface loss, which can lead to increased dentin hypersensitivity in patients. Dentin exposure raises the chance of tooth sensitivity.
8. Women who are pregnant or nursing: Studies evaluating bleaching chemicals, for example, do not often enrol pregnant patients. This population has as far not been the subject of any investigation. So far, research has failed to establish whether bleaching teeth during pregnancy is safe or not. Pregnant or nursing women should always wait to get therapy as a safety measure.
9. When the cementum or dentin covering the teeth's, roots become exposed, the likelihood of tooth sensitivity rises.
10. Teeth with extensive caries: Active dental caries that may be close to the pulp should be given special attention. The mineral loss in caries lesions results in the formation and growth of porosities which act as diffusion pathways for bleaching agent into the pulp chamber and can lead to pulpal inflammation. These problems need to be temporarily treated prior to the whitening treatment and finalized once the colour is stabilized.

There are a lot of different whitener strategies detailed in books and online. Many approaches are available, each utilizing a unique combination of whitening chemicals, concentrations, application periods, modes, and light activation techniques.

However, three fundamental bleaching approaches exist.

1) At-home or Dentist-supervised night guard bleaching
2) In-office or power bleaching
3) Bleaching with over–the-counter bleaching products.

At-home or dentist supervised night-guard bleaching contains a small amount of bleaching chemical (3.5-6.5% hydrogen peroxide, or 10-20% carbamide peroxide). During follow-up appointments, the dentist watches while the patient does the treatment on their own. This method has been around for a long time and is one of the most used ones.

In-office bleaching generally uses a hydrogen peroxide solution ranging from 25% to 35% in concentration to whiten teeth. In this method, the dentist has full command of the whitening process and may stop it as soon as the patient reaches the desired shade or effect. After the gums and cheeks are protected, the whitening gel is applied to the teeth. Peroxide can be further activated by using heat or light.

Over-the-counter beaching things that have grown in demand over the past few years. These solutions are designed to be self-applied to the teeth using gum shields, strips, or paint-on formulations. They contain a low concentration of hydrogen peroxide, often ranging from 3-6%.

At-Home Bleaching or Night-Guard Vital Tooth Bleaching

The most popular, predictable and well-researched method of bleaching teeth are Night Guard Vital Bleaching. This technique was developed by Haywood and Heymann in 1989. Bleaching with a night guard, either at home or under a dentist's supervision, entails using a weak whitening chemical (10-20% carbamide peroxide, or 3.5-6.5% hydrogen peroxide). In most cases, the suggested dosages of carbamide peroxide are 10% for 8 hours per day and 15-20% for 3-4 hours per day. Patients do this therapy on their own, however dentists should be present at follow-up appointments to ensure proper supervision. This technique is often supplemented by a heat or a light source to enhance the action of peroxide. The technique is accomplished without the anaesthesia to determine the patient's pain threshold for the heat level. In contemporary aesthetic dentistry, at-home tooth bleaching has emerged as one of the most widely adopted, conservative interventions for improving tooth colour. This approach offers patients the convenience of performing whitening procedures within the comfort of their own homes, under professional supervision. Unlike in-office bleaching, which typically utilizes higher concentrations of bleaching agents and requires chairside administration, at-home bleaching relies on lower concentrations of peroxide-based agents applied over extended periods. This modality has gained popularity due to its cost-effectiveness, reduced chair time, and the ability to maintain gradual and controlled colour improvement. The principles underpinning at-home bleaching involve the diffusion of peroxide-based oxidizing agents through the enamel and dentin, leading to oxidative modification of chromophores and consequent colour lightening. Understanding the chemical, biological, and clinical aspects of at-home bleaching is essential for optimizing outcomes while minimizing potential adverse effects.

Carbamide peroxide and hydrogen peroxide are the two most common chemical agents used for teeth whitening when done at home. When carbamide peroxide, a combination of urea and hydrogen peroxide, breaks down in water, it releases about a third of the hydrogen peroxide and urea that it originally contained. The gradual release of hydrogen peroxide ensures sustained oxidative activity over extended periods, making carbamide peroxide suitable for overnight or extended wear applications, such as in custom-fitted trays. Hydrogen peroxide, in contrast, may be utilized directly in lower concentrations for at-home use, but carbamide peroxide remains preferred due to its controlled release profile and lower associated sensitivity risk.

Using hydrogen peroxide as an oxidizing agent in oxidation-reduction processes is the main way bleaching works. Hydrogen peroxide, when placed on teeth, breaks down the tooth's protective enamel and dentin, creating free radicals such hydroxyl (•OH) and perhydroxyl (HO_2•) radicals, which are part of the reactive oxygen species (ROS). Chromophore molecules have conjugated double bonds that these radicals may cleave, resulting in the breakdown of large pigmented complexes into smaller, less coloured bits. The disruption of these chromophoric structures reduces the molecules' capacity to absorb visible light, thereby resulting in tooth whitening. The efficacy of peroxide-based bleaching is influenced by numerous factors, including pH, temperature, light exposure, and the presence of catalytic metals, which may accelerate the decomposition of peroxide into active radicals.

Mechanisms of Colour Change

The molecular mechanisms underlying at-home bleaching involve oxidative modification of chromophore molecules embedded within the enamel and dentin. Chromophores typically consist of conjugated double bonds or aromatic rings, which absorb visible light and impart colour to the tooth. Hydrogen peroxide and its reactive derivatives oxidize these chromophores through cleavage of double bonds, ring-opening reactions, or oxidation of associated functional groups. The resulting smaller molecules possess altered electronic structures that do not absorb visible light as efficiently, thereby producing a whiter appearance. The diffusion of peroxide through enamel prisms and dentinal tubules allows bleaching to affect both superficial and deeper intrinsic discolorations.

Advantages and Disadvantages of Home Whitening

ADVANTAGES:

1. Simple, self-administered method for patient to be used,
2. Simple for dentists to monitor,
3. Less chair time and cost effective,
4. Patient can bleach their teeth at their convenience,
5. High degree of safety.

DISADVANTAGES:

1. Patients' compliance is mandatory
2. Colour change is dependent on diligence of use. (Leonard et al 2003)
3. Chances of abuse by using excessive amount of bleach for too many hours per day

Factors That Guard the Prognosis of Home Bleaching

1. History or presence of sensitive teeth
2. Extremely dark gingival third of tooth visible during smiling
3. Extensive white spots
4. Translucent teeth
5. Excessive gingival recession and exposed root surfaces.

Protocol For Bleaching

The protocol for night guard vital tooth bleaching is based on that development by Haywood and Heymann 1989.

- The patient's medical history is carefully reviewed, a thorough physical examination is performed, and a differential diagnosis is made to determine the source of the discoloration.
- Records are kept of restorations in both the target and neighbouring teeth. Bleaching will not alter the colour of veneers, crowns, or other existing restorations; thus, they are marked in the chart.
- The periodontal tissue thickness and any pockets are documented.
- Using a three-way syringe, the teeth that are to be bleached are exposed to air while any sensitivity is noted. Every tooth, but especially the one that was already sensitive before the whitening process, will be more sensitive thereafter. The patient should be informed of this.
- Instead of bleaching for an entire night, those who are diagnosed with sensitivity early may just need to apply it for two hours at a time.
- Tooth surface loss caused by, in particular, erosion may be sensitive and becomes more sensitive after bleaching procedure so, such defects should be well recorded during the history taking.
- The patient and the dentist agree on the tooth shade using a value-oriented (light to dark) shade guide. Before beginning the bleaching operation, we make note of this hue and also provide the patient with a written record.
- It is important to consult with the patient about the possibility of whitening only one arch instead of both.
- It is important to document any irregularities in the tooth enamel or dentine, the amount and quality of restorations, and the existence or absence of periodontal disease.
- Radiographs, before the initiation of the procedure should be well recorded and diagnosed of any periodontal radiolucency or abnormalities, any pulpal atypical morphology, sclerosis etc.

- A preoperative photograph of the teeth and the opposing teeth to be bleached is taken, with a reference from the shade tab held parallel to the tooth to be bleached.
- Patients should be made aware of the shades (light or dark) of the already existing restorations, crowns, bridges, implant abutments, veneers present in the mouth and possible shade changes in accordance to these restorations.

Clinical Procedure

Initial consultation

- The advantages and disadvantages of tooth whitening.
- Alternatives to whitening treatments.
- Any side effects that may be experienced (such as sensitivity, gingival irritation).
- The risks and benefits of the procedures; the patient's informed consent should be obtained.
- All treatment options, including the possibility that more than one whitening treatment may need to be undertaken.
- The duration of treatment.

Clinical examination of all teeth

- It is important to do a thorough assessment of the patient's oral health, including their soft tissues, mucosa, teeth, and gingiva.
- Inspect the current repairs for damage.
- Look for signs of dental disease and periapical radiolucency in your most recent radiographs.
- Using radiographs, one may determine the sensitivity levels by gauging the size and health of the tooth pulps.

Planning of the treatment

- For the sake of the patient's ability to make an informed comparison, it is recommended to whiten only one arch at a time.

- Pictures are shot using the shade option that corresponds to the teeth as they are right now. It is also possible to take images within the mouth.
- It is also essential to discuss with patients that their existing composite restorations may not match after whitening and that it may be necessary to replace these composites with lighter ones after the whitening procedures.

Impression taking

- Taking high-quality imprints that mimic the shape and size of the teeth's surfaces is essential. You can use alginate or any other precise substance. Keep the air bubbles from building up and showing up as positives on the cast.

Preparation of the cast and fabrication of the tray

- To avoid cast distortion, alginate impressions should be poured and cast as soon as possible. For the plaster cast to be strong enough, it should be horseshoe shaped and substantial in size.

Placement of block out resin

- The teeth to be bleached are identified on the cast. Gently place the block-out material in the middle of each tooth.
- In most cases, the buccal sides of the cast teeth are where the block-out material that is utilized to make the reservoirs is applied.

Apply separator/cold mould seal

- After the cast is made, a cold-mould seal is applied. The vacuum-formed thermoplastic material will be easier to remove in this way.

Choose the tray sheet material and tray design

Tray material

- When it comes to trays, ethyl vinyl acetate is by far the most popular material. There is a wide range of thicknesses available for EVA, a flexible substance.
- The most popular thickness is 0.035 inch, while thinner options are available at 0.02 inch and thicker ones are available at 0.05 inch for individuals who suffer from bruxism.
- It is important that the tray material be sturdy, non-allergic, and easy to clean.
- The material may be readily modified and treated to a smooth edge, protecting the tongue and gingiva from harm.

Tray design

- To ensure a successful whitening treatment and patient compliance, it is crucial that the whitening tray is designed, constructed, and fits properly.
- The tray is designed to keep the bleaching gel in place while the teeth are being bleached. If the tray is not well-designed or -made, it will not achieve the desired result.
- The individual issue at hand, the kind and extent of the discolouration, and the available designs will dictate the approach taken.
- A variety of tray designs exist.

  Tray with Reservoirs: An empty area that has been made in the teeth-whitening tray is called a reservoir. Another name for the reservoir is a spacer. In order to keep the whitening solution in the tray and in touch with the teeth for an extended length of time, the reservoir within the tray serves as a container for the substance. In order to create the reservoir, the buccal surfaces of the teeth on the plaster model are coated with light-cured composite resin.

It is important to design the tray so as to avoid gel coming into contact with soft tissues. the reservoirs allow per-hydroxyl ions released from the Carbamide peroxide to contact the darkest discoloured areas of the teeth.
The filled tray can seat more securely on teeth thanks to the reservoirs. In most cases, the tray will be too short at the gum line if it does not sit correctly. The bleaching of the teeth's neck may not be effective as a consequence. The unprotected gel can react with salivary peroxidases and catalase, quickly inactivating the hydrogen peroxide.
The reservoir can be of different sizes, depending on specific conditions.

a) The Bulbous and darker teeth require greater reservoir space.

b) For bleaching neck of the teeth reservoir should extend over the gingival margins so that they are capable of holding the gel in cervical margin and do not pinch the soft tissues.
Trays with no reservoirs: Recent research has disproved the long-held belief that dental whitening trays with reservoirs are essential for effective results. Better tray retention and less material usage per application are two benefits of this method. The whitening substance may be compressed against the tooth surface and penetrated more effectively and faster using a tray that fits the teeth better.

Scalloped Trays: Trays with scalloped edges minimize touch with delicate tissues. Because of how little whitening agent they utilize, they irritate the gums very little. The gingival margins are followed by the tray. Once the tray material is customized to fit the model, the labial portion of the transparent tray may be utilized to delineate the gingival boundaries using a permanent ink pen. After taking the tray out, you may cut following the contour with a smooth edge that the tongue will have no problem with. The gingival tissues may be exposed to some extruded gel if the scalloping is placed below the gingival boundary.

Straight-line Trays: These trays are cut out 2 mm over the labial incisors. Touati et al. (1999) suggest this particular tray for your needs. According to them, this design outshines the anatomic tray design in terms of ease of use, ease of implementation, little stress to the surrounding oral tissues, and quality of border seal. Each tooth has a thin reservoir in the centre and the interproximal gaps are filled in with this design.

Single-tooth Trays: Single-tooth trays are designed to bleach individual teeth. A standard tray is adjusted by trimming it away from the labial aspect of the adjacent teeth. By cutting the tray salivary enzymes inactivate any hydrogen peroxide coming in contact with the adjacent teeth. This is important for single dark tooth bleaching.

Combination Trays: If a regular tray does not hold the gel over the specific teeth you need to treat, a combination tray can be adapted to do the trick. A less sturdy and less retentive tray is the result of cutting windows. To ensure retention, these trays should be extended into the premolar and molar areas' natural undercuts. Cast the plastic in the vacuum tray-forming machine The occlusal side of the modified cast should be facing the plastic sheet when it is put on the platform. A vacuum-forming machine is used to conform the thermoplastic material to the mould after it has been heated till it turns transparent. Prior to trimming the trays, make sure the plastic has cooled down enough to prevent deformation. Sharp scissors or a scalpel is used to remove excess material.

Finishing and polishing of the tray

Once you reach around 1 cm above the gingival margin, continue to cut the tray with scissors. To ensure that no rough spots remain, use a soft cotton wheel to perform the final finishing and polishing of the edges.

Fitting of the tray

- The tray's fit is verified. Blanching the delicate tissues could harm the gums, thus it is best to avoid it. Therefore, it is important to have the patient use their tongue to feel for any sore spots.
- Teeth to be bleached should be marked with a permanent ink pen for easy identification of the patient while placing the bleaching gel at home.
- Shade should be well confirmed with the reference value- oriented shade guide.
- Patients are provided with printed instructions and a about 10% carbamide peroxide solution.
- The patient should be given a suitable box, similar to an orthodontic retainer, to keep the bleaching tray in when it is not in use.
- It is recommended to provide 5% potassium nitrate ($KNO3$) to patients who have sensitivity. Either use it two weeks before bleaching, or put it in a tray and wear it for thirty minutes before each bleaching treatment.

Instructions For the Patients for The Use Of 10% Carbamide Peroxide

- Brush your teeth thoroughly in the normal fashion
- As usual, brush your teeth completely.
- Take the syringe tip off the 10% carbamide peroxide gel and inject a little amount into the tray, making sure to push it towards the front and deeper areas of each tooth's mould. This will help with the bleaching process.
- Set the gel aside in the
- Seat the tray over the teeth and slowly press down firmly.

- A finger, a tissue, or a soft toothbrush should be used to remove excess gel that will flow beyond the edge of the tray.
- Rinse gently- do not swallow. The tray is usually worn overnight but as long as it is worn for 2 hours the process is effective enough to show desired results.
- In morning remove the tray and brush residual gel from the teeth, remove gel from tray as well clean thoroughly and keep in a safe container.
- Do not eat drink or smoke while wearing the bleaching tray.
- Carbamide peroxide should not be exposed to heat, sunlight or extreme cold.
- Comparative Analysis with In-Office Bleaching

While in-office bleaching procedures utilize higher concentrations of peroxide and may provide rapid results within a single session, at-home bleaching offers a safer and more gradual approach. Clinical studies indicate that the final whitening outcome achieved with at-home bleaching is comparable to in-office protocols when proper compliance is maintained. Furthermore, at-home bleaching allows patients to adjust treatment duration based on tolerance, making it particularly suitable for individuals with sensitive teeth or high aesthetic demands.

- Recent Advances in At-Home Bleaching

Recent research in at-home bleaching has focused on optimizing peroxide formulations, reducing sensitivity, and enhancing diffusion into dental tissues. The incorporation of desensitizing agents, such as potassium nitrate or fluoride, into bleaching gels has been shown to mitigate transient sensitivity while maintaining efficacy. Additionally, novel delivery systems, including pre-filled disposable trays, flexible thermoplastic trays, and microencapsulated peroxide gels, have been developed to improve patient convenience, safety, and compliance. Investigations into the synergistic use of low-intensity light or chemical activators to accelerate peroxide release are ongoing, although their clinical significance in at-home settings remains under study.

- Long-Term Considerations

Long-term considerations in at-home bleaching include the maintenance of colour stability and prevention of relapse. The effectiveness of at-home bleaching may gradually diminish over months due to exposure to chromogenic substances, aging of enamel and dentin, and lifestyle habits. Maintenance protocols typically involve periodic repeat applications of low-concentration peroxide, often for one or two nights per month, to preserve the achieved whitening effect. Regular dental evaluations are essential to monitor enamel health, assess for new restorations, and provide professional prophylaxis that supports aesthetic outcomes.

Emerging technologies in at-home bleaching aim to enhance efficacy, reduce treatment times, and minimize sensitivity. Research is ongoing into the development of peroxide-free bleaching agents utilizing alternative oxidizing compounds, enzymes, or nanoparticle delivery systems that can target chromophores more selectively. Furthermore, the integration of digital technologies, such as 3D-printed trays, customized dosing, and telemonitoring of patient compliance, has the potential to revolutionize at-home bleaching protocols, providing precision treatment tailored to individual dental morphology and patient preferences.

At-home tooth bleaching represents a safe, effective, and patient-centred approach to achieving aesthetic improvement in tooth colour. By utilizing low-concentration peroxide agents delivered through custom-fitted trays, patients can achieve gradual and controlled whitening while minimizing adverse effects such as sensitivity and gingival irritation. The chemical principles underlying at-home bleaching, including oxidative cleavage of chromophores and diffusion of peroxide through enamel and dentin, are well-established and supported by extensive clinical research. Adherence to proper protocols, patient education, and periodic professional follow-up are essential to optimizing outcomes and maintaining long-term results. With ongoing advancements in formulation, delivery systems, and technology, at-home bleaching is poised to remain a cornerstone of conservative aesthetic dentistry, providing patients with predictable, safe, and convenient options for enhancing their smiles.

In-Office or Power Bleaching

It was Harlan in 1884 who allegedly used hydrogen peroxide for the first time to whiten teeth. "Hydrogen dioxide" was the name he gave to hydrogen peroxide. It was Prinz who initially utilized it in 1910 for both vital and non-vital teeth. In 1918, Abbot once again improved bleaching efficiency by combining high-intensity light with hydrogen peroxide.

High concentration bleaching materials, with or without light, are harmful to soft tissues and cause sensitivity-related issues, despite the fact that chair-side treatment time is decreased.

Mechanism

The discolouring molecules contain sequential conjugated double bonds that must be broken down by the hydrogen peroxide. For this, hydrogen peroxide has to continuously release per-hydroxyl ions while the material is kept away from soft tissues.

Technique For In-Office Bleaching

- Patient's assessment:

Before starting the bleaching procedure, a detailed history of the patient is recorded and the proper treatment protocol should be planned for the patient. Pre-operative photographs, sensitivity history, shade selection, bleaching technique and material and cost should be decided well in advance before initiating the treatment and explained to the patient.

- Isolation of teeth:

Soft tissues should be protected throughout the bleaching procedure when applying high- concentration hydrogen peroxide gel.

To make sure the tooth necks get bleached, you need to put the teeth in the rubber dam and then flip it over into the gingival sulcus.

- Rubber dam application

Since the cervical margins are notoriously difficult to isolate, it is wise to put an additional layer of protective caulk (Oraseal, Ultradent Product Inc.) beneath the dam. Prior to using bleaching gel, make sure to remove any caulking material that may have gotten onto the tooth surface. To secure the rubber dam in place, floss ligatures can be wound around the tooth necks. Dental floss that has been waxed is required for the ligatures. The hydrogen peroxide gel may be drawn up by capillary action using unswollen dental floss, which acts as a wick, resulting in burns to the gingival tissues. Placement of rubber dam and inversion of the dam into the gingival cervices is not pleasant and sometimes can be painful for the patients.

- Bleaching Material

Because it is a thick gel, the bleaching agent does not run off the teeth and is easy to apply and position precisely. The contents of two tubes are mixed together by squeezing the material from one tube to the other until the two tubes are entirely interlocked; this is one method of distribution for a 38% hydrogen peroxide gel. Because of the gel's red colour, the operator can easily see where the gel is going and how to apply it. The recommended consumption time for the blended gel is 10 days. It is important to keep high concentration bleaching gels refrigerated since they become unstable when exposed to changes in temperature. The material's shelf life depends on this.

- Application Of the Bleaching Material

All of the teeth that need whitening are coated simultaneously with the gel, which typically comprises hydrogen peroxide and carbamide peroxide, and kept in place for around fifteen minutes. The gel has to be stirred. To make it go more quickly, you can add heat or light. At fifteen-minute intervals, you will need to rinse off the gel, dry your teeth, and apply fresh bleaching solution. The easiest approach to remove most of the gel with minimal splashing is to use high-volume aspiration. The process must be carried out three or four times. Consequently, it is wise to allocate around 90 minutes for chair-side time.

- Acceleration techniques

Acceleration of chair-side bleaching can be attempted in various ways.

1. Increasing the concentration of the hydrogen peroxide: Oxidation occurs more rapidly with increasing concentrations of hydrogen peroxide. Hydrogen peroxide concentrations between 25% and 38% are often regarded as excessive. As a result, patients and dental staff may have heightened sensitivity, necessitating further measures to isolate and protect themselves.
2. Use of Light-activated Catalyst: Bleaching materials often have light-activated catalysts added to them so that the process may be controlled when it is triggered. Light is utilized to start the catalytic reaction after the item is in the proper place.
3. Use of Heat and Light: When the hydrogen peroxide gel is heated, it dissociates more quickly, releasing more per-hydroxyl ions that can break down the tooth discoloration molecules. The rate of dissociation of hydrogen peroxide is doubled for every 10-degree rise.

It is important to not anaesthetise teeth when heat is applied to the teeth, so that patient can report of any discomfort caused due to increased temperature.

- Concentration and Efficacy

Because the teeth are separated beneath a rubber dam during chair-side whitening, they quickly become lighter as a result of dehydration. The bleaching time of a hydrogen peroxide gel is directly proportional to its concentration. If you apply a high concentration under a rubber dam, the dehydration effect can be more pronounced, and the teeth might "rebound" in colour, becoming darker as they rehydrate.

Bleaching does not remove but lightens the surface coating and deposits which gives rise to discolouration, by bleaching. Superficial stains like tobacco, coffee or other highly coloured substances are easily bleached but better managed by oral prophylaxis scaling and polishing.

Although night guard essential bleaching is great at removing discoloration caused by simple chemicals, it takes much longer to break down more complicated compounds, such as benzene rings and metal ions with sequential conjugated double bonds in teeth.

Up to three or four visits are required in case of in-office chair side power bleaching to obtain a similar result as evident in case of night-guard vital bleaching. protocols is necessary to preserve enamel integrity.

CHAPTER 9

NON-VITAL TOOTH BLEACHING

DR. NEHA VERMA

To eliminate discoloration, chemical agents are used within the coronal section of teeth that have undergone endodontic treatment; this process is known as intra-coronal bleaching (American association of endodontics 2010).

INDICATIONS:

- Discoloration of pulp chamber
- Dentine discoloration
- Discolorations not amenable to extra coronal bleaching
- Adequate root canal treatment has been performed

CONTRAINDICATIONS:

- Superficial enamel discolouration
- Defective enamel formation
- Severe dentine loss
- Presence of caries
- Discoloured restorations

Bleaching Agents for Whitening of Root Filled Teeth

Hydrogen peroxide, carbamide peroxide, and sodium perborate are the most popular bleaching chemicals used to whiten teeth that have had root canal treatment.

Sodium perborate in the form of mono, tri-, or tetrahydrate is used as a H2O2 releasing agent. The whitening efficacy of sodium perborate mono-, tri-, or tetrahydrate mixture with either water or hydrogen peroxide is not different. H2O2 is released during the decomposition of perborate. Several factors, including pH, light, temperature, co-catalysts, and metallic reaction partners, can cause the released H2O2 to produce various radicals or ions (Feinman et al. 1991, Goldstein & Garber 1995). Long, coloured molecules can have their double bonds broken by radicals, or metallic oxides, such as Fe2O3 (Fe3+), can be reduced to the colourless form of FeO (Fe3+).

Clinical Bleaching Techniques for Endodontically Treated Teeth

Bleaching of endodontically treated teeth that present with chromatic alterations is a conservative alternative to a more invasive aesthetic treatment such as placement of crowns or veneers.

Preliminary treatment:

It is important to determine the cause of tooth discolouration.

- To find out how bad the discoloration is on the outside, you should clean the tooth's surface first.
- It is important to keep the patient aware about what to expect from the whitening process and that there is no assurance that their teeth will return to their original colour after treatment.
- In addition, details on the steps to take, potential risks, and how often to use the bleaching chemical for best results should be included.
- Document the progress made by taking pictures before and after the therapy so the patient can see the final product.
- To ensure the root filling is of good quality, a radiograph should be taken before therapy. Not only should it stop microbes from seeping from the coronal to the apical area, but it should also stop the bleaching chemical from reaching the apical tissue and damaging it.
- Therefore, an inadequate root filling should be replaced and the new filling should be placed and allowed to set for at least 7 days before starting with the bleaching procedure.
- Rubber dam isolation to isolate the tooth, to prevent re-infection of root canal, and to prevent the adjacent structure from bleaching agent.

Different types of intracoronal bleaching

1. Walking bleach technique
2. Thermo-catalytic technique
3. In-office bleaching technique
4. Inside-outside bleaching

Walking Bleach Technique

The 1st Salvas published Marsh's account of the walking bleach procedure, which involves mixing sodium perborate with distilled water. The treatment involved leaving the mixture in the pulp area and sealing the access cavity with temporary cement for a duration of 7 days. Spasser reevaluated and adjusted the sodium perborate and water combination. in an effort to increase the mixture's bleaching efficacy, Nutting & Poe suggested substituting 30% hydrogen peroxide for water. Intracoronal bleaching with the same combination is still going strong today.

Preparation of the pulp cavity:

- Before preparation of the pulp cavity rubber dam isolation is must.
- Cleaning of the pulp cavity with sodium hypochlorite is recommended.
- To eliminate the smear layer and open the dentinal tubules, it may be advised to treat the dentine of the access cavity with 37% orthophosphoric acid in some circumstances. Because the bleaching chemical may now reach deeper into the opening tubules of the dentin, the bleaching action is enhanced. This is a contentious idea, though.

Cervical Seal:

- With the use of Gates-Glidden or large burs, the root filling should be lowered 1-2mm below the CEJ.
- Remove any debris or residues of endodontic materials from the surface of the cavity.

- Root fillings are insufficient to stop the bleaching agent from diffusing from the pulp chamber to the apical foramen. You will need a BASE, such as GIC, IRM (interim restorative material), resin composite, zinc oxide eugenol, zinc phosphate cement, etc., to stop the bleaching agent from penetrating the root canals.

Application of Bleaching Agent:

Intracoronal bleaching is best accomplished with a 2:1 (g/ml) mixture of sodium perborate (tetrahydrate) and purified water. Applying 3% hydrogen peroxide may be necessary for really discoloured areas. It is recommended to change the bleaching chemical every 3-7 days using an amalgam carrier or plugger. If the discoloration is severe, it may take 2-4 sessions before you may see any results from the bleaching. In order to avoid "over-whitening," patients should be advised to check the tooth colour every day.

Temporary Filling:

To achieve a temporary adhesive filling, etch the enamel edges of the cavity with 37% orthophosphoric acid before applying the bleaching agent. To guarantee the efficacy of the walking bleach technique and to prevent the bleaching substance from leaking into the oral cavity, a resin composite sound barrier surrounding the access cavity is necessary.

To make it easier to insert filling material over a soft bleaching agent, a sterile cotton pellet that has been impregnated with dentine bonding agent can be placed on top of the bleaching agent and then light-cured. The enamel edges of the access cavity are the only places the temporary filling should be applied.

Thermocatalytic Technique

In this method, a pulp chamber containing 30–35% hydrogen peroxide is heated using an electric heating equipment or specialized lamps.

Various commercial heat applicators, such as heated metal instruments, can be used to apply heat. At each session, you will change the pellet with a "fresh" bleaching ingredient and apply heat three or four times. Foam and the release of oxygen from the preparation are byproducts of a process that occurs when heat is applied. Like with the walking bleach method, the pulp chamber is shut off after each session so that the bleaching chemical may continue to work between visits.

In- office technique: The process of externally whitening teeth that have had root canal treatment using hydrogen peroxide or carbamide peroxide gels at high concentrations (15%-35%). A bleaching tray is used to apply the whitening gel directly to the tooth, which is covered with a rubber dam and does not have an access hole. Some people thought that in order for the bleaching gel to reach the discoloured tooth, the pulp chamber needed be open while the tooth was being bleached. Here, a bleaching tray is used to apply the whitening gel to the pulp chamber and buccal surfaces through the access hole.

This method is not without its dangers, since germs and stains can get into dentin through an unprotected access hole. Bacterial permeation of the tooth is still detectable, even after a successful root canal treatment. Since this is the case, the root filling should be securely fastened at the opening using a restorative substance like resin composite or glass-ionomer cement. The in-office procedures can also be used when the walking bleach technique does not produce satisfactory results after 3-4 applications.

The inside-outside bleaching technique: The term "interior/external bleaching" might describe this process as well. The Modified Walking Bleaching Technique and Patient-Administered Intracoronal Bleaching Technique are alternative names for the same procedure (Liebenberg 1997). This method integrates the intra-coronal bleaching procedure with the at-home bleaching method. Bleaching material, typically 10% carbamide peroxide, is introduced into the pulp chamber through an open access cavity that is left after barrier replacement. Placing the bleaching tray on the tooth helps to keep the material in place. So, it is possible to bleach inside and externally simultaneously.

Indications:

- Treatment for adolescents with incomplete gingival maturations

- A single dark non-vital tooth where the surrounding teeth are sufficiently light.

Procedure:

Preparation of barrier: The availability of a satisfactory root canal treatment and the lack of apical disease are confirmed by a pre-operative X-ray. The tooth is prepared for the current extra-coronal repair by isolating it with a rubber dam. Gutta percha is removed to a depth of 2-3mm below the cement-epithelial junction, much as in the intra-coronal procedure. Making room for the barrier is the goal of gutta percha removal. The gutta percha is covered with a protective barrier so that the bleach does not leak into the root canal system through the cemento-enamel junction. As a barrier, you can use either resin-modified glass ionomer or traditional glass ionomer cement. Some have recommended covering the exposed gutta percha with a calcium hydroxide plug that is about 1mm thick. These preventative measures are designed to keep the medium at an alkaline pH. Since a decrease in pH at the cervical level has been linked to cervical resorption, this explains the phenomenon. A periapical radiograph can be taken at this stage to check whether barrier has been well placed, but this is not mandatory.

Cleaning the access cavity: All pulp horn remnants are extracted and the access cavity is thoroughly cleansed. It is sufficient to etch the inside surface of the access cavity in order to clean it. It has no effect in enhancing bleaching. Put a cotton wool pellet in the access hole so food does not pack into it.

Shade assessment: The pre-operative shade is taken both of the non-vital colour and the surrounding teeth and noted down.

Instructions for home bleaching: Make sure the bleaching tray is comfortable and fits properly. During therapy, the patient is asked not to bite with their front teeth. The patient will receive sufficient bleaching supplies and instructions before being sent home. Prior to bleaching, the cotton pellet in the access cavity is removed using the tooth pick. You have two options: either fill the open chamber with bleaching solution from the syringe before placing the bleaching tray inside, or fill the tray with more bleaching material and place it in the gap between the teeth that have an open chamber. The tooth is rinsed with water from a syringe after the bleaching procedure, and then new cotton wool is placed back into the tooth. After eating, the tooth is rinsed with water once again to remove any food particles, and a new cotton wool pellet is placed back into the canal.

Treatment Timings: If a patient can change the solutions every two hours, 5 to 8 applications are enough so as to achieve a desired whitening of the teeth. Unless the tooth discoloration is really severe, it is recommended to apply the bleaching agent throughout the day for greater control over the lightening process.

Reassessment of the shade and bleaching results: When patient returns in 3-7 days shade changes are assessed. If sufficient lightening has occurred the bleaching procedure may be terminated.

Sealing the access cavity: The next step is to apply a temporary bandage to close the access cavity. Two weeks must elapse before the final restoration can be placed so that the tooth may expel its oxygen and the enamel or composite can strengthen its binding. You can use a spongy pellet to administer catalase or sodium ascorbate into the access cavity for three minutes if waiting two weeks before inserting the final repair is not feasible. By hastening the breakdown of hydrogen peroxide into oxygen and water, catalase eliminates any dormant hydrogen peroxide. To begin, sodium hypochlorite is irrigated into the access cavity to remove any residual material. Once the access cavity is cleansed, catalase can be used. Dentine in the pulp chamber, enamel around the access cavity, and the cavo-surface edges are etched for 15 seconds using 37% phosphoric acid. The next step is to use chemicals that bind the teeth. It has been demonstrated that bonding agents including acetone can counteract the effects of the acid erosion on the strength of the enamel cuticle. The composite repair is applied to the access cavity in layers, with a flowable layer at the bottom and incremental builds of composite, before covering the glass ionomer.

Review: The tooth should be periodically reviewed and a radiograph taken annually to check for any signs of cervical inflammatory response.

Benefits of inside/outside bleaching technique:

- There is a greater surface area on both the inside and the outside that bleach may reach.
- Bleach with a neutral pH and a lower concentration of 10% carbamide peroxide is utilized.
- The goal of this method is to prevent cervical resorption as much as possible.
- By leaving the access cavity accessible, the need to change the dressing is removed. It used to be common for the oxygen produced during bleaching to loosen the temporary dressing and cause it to fall off the tooth. No pressure buildup occurs, and oxygen may leave in a natural way.
- Time required for treatment is cut down from weeks to days.
- Once the appropriate colour is obtained, the patient can stop filling the pulp.
- To remove any remaining oxygen, use catalase before placing the repair.
- Activating bleaching material does not need heat.

Risks:

- Potential for cervical resorption is reduced but still exists.
- The tooth could be over bleached through over-zealous application of the bleaching material by the patient.

Prognosis of non-vital bleached teeth:

The ideal first outcome of bleaching, according to certain in-vivo and in-vitro research, is for the bleached tooth or teeth to match the colour of the neighbouring tooth or teeth exactly. On rare occasions, however, you may notice a darkening of the tooth's enamel following internal bleaching. This is likely due to the spread of germs and staining chemicals through the tiny spaces between the filling and tooth.

The outlook for discoloration brought on by restoration materials is uncertain. Bleach has a very low efficacy against several metal ions, including mercury, silver, copper, and iodine. In contrast to teeth discoloured due to medications or restorations, which are more difficult to bleach, trauma or necrosis-induced discoloration may be effectively bleached in around 95% of instances, according to Brown. There is a difference in opinion as to whether teeth that respond rapidly to bleaching have a better long term colour stability prognosis. Some studied have reported that stained teeth in young patients are easier to bleach than discolouration in older patients.

Other Options for Nonvital Teeth

Combination of Power and Home Bleaching Treatments

Motivating patients to follow the home bleaching treatment and keep bleaching at home is a common goal of this strategy. Typically, one or two sessions of power bleaching are performed in the office. The next step is to provide the patient with the necessary materials and the home bleaching instructions tray so they can complete the process at home.

Matrix bleaching at home with a weaker hydrogen peroxide or carbamide peroxide reagent follows an initial 30 minutes of power bleaching with 35 to 50% supersaturated hydrogen peroxide. Just thirty to forty-five minutes throughout the night is the matrix system turned on.

Benefits of this combination treatment are:

- The monotony of making many trips to the doctor and applying rubber dams is rendered obsolete; now, a single application is required.
- It lessens the cost of lengthy doctor's appointments.
- While the tray is being created, power bleaching gives it a boost and shows that it is improving.

CHAPTER 10

BLEACHING AND MICROABRASION

DR. NEHA VERMA

Enamel micro-abrasion is a procedure in which a microscopic layer of enamel is simultaneously eroded and abraded with a special compound leaving a perfectly intact enamel surface behind. It is used to treat enamel discolorations which may be the result of hypermineralizations, hypominearlizations or staining. Croll (1991) called the process 'Enamel Demineralization'.

Micro abrasion technique can be used in combination with home bleaching or power bleaching to remove these discolorations more effectively but which procedure is done first depends on the specific case. The microabrasion techniques can be undertaken in patients of all ages: adolescents, adults, and the elderly.

Micro abrasion enhances tooth colour by erasing the surface discoloured enamel, which is different from bleaching. The removal of discoloration is a permanent process. When a specific isolated surface discoloration is present but a change in tooth colour is not necessary, micro-abrasion is the method of choice.

Tooth bleaching lightens, whitens, and brightens teeth, which enhances their colour. In contrast to micro abrasion, bleaching leaves the tooth's form and the enamel's protective coating of fluoride intact. Teeth may gradually deepen in tone over the years, but they will never be the same dark shade again.

Sometimes, following micro abrasion, the tooth seems more yellow or darker, although the two methods can be utilized in conjunction with each other. Thus, to enhance tooth colour, bleaching can be applied after microabrasion. Combining treatments yields the greatest outcomes and improvements.

Indications:

- Developmental intrinsic stains and discolorations
- Superficial surface enamel stains
- Yellow-brown areas
- Multi-coloured stains
- Areas of enamel fluorosis
- White patches, white spots
- Irregular surface textures

Contraindications:

- Age related staining
- Tetracycline staining
- Deep enamel hypoplastic lesions
- Amelogenesis Imperfecta
- Dentinogenesis lesions
- Areas of deep enamel and dentine stains

Evolution of the Technique

Several microabrasion methods have been detailed for enhancing the aesthetics of fluorotic teeth. Using a combination of 36% HCl acid and heat, Dr. Walter Kane (1916) successfully treated enamel fluorosis stains. The acid was applied to the modified enamel using a hot metallic tool to enhance its penetration and speed up the acid-enamel chemical reaction. Fearing for the method's safety, Raper et al. recommended 18% hydrochloric acid applied and massaged with a cotton-wrapped wooden spatula for no more than 10 minutes.

Mechanical application with a low rotation micromotor was indicated in the 1960s, McInnes used a mixture of five parts of 36% hydrochloric acid, or HCl; five parts of 30% hydrogen peroxide; and one part of ether as a topical treatment. This solution was further modified with 20% sodium hydroxide instead of 36% hydrochloric acid.40 Since sodium hydroxide is highly Alkaline in nature, it dissolves calcium of the enamel at a slower rate.

Hence, modified McInnes solution is considered to be a slower but safer alternative to McInness solution. In 1984, McCloskey reported the use of 18% hydrochloric acid swabbed on teeth for the removal of superficial fluorosis stains. Subsequently, in 1986, Croll and Cavanaugh modified the technique to include the use of pumice with hydrochloric acid to form a paste applied with a tongue blade. It involves the surface dissolution of the enamel by acid along with the abrasiveness of the pumice to remove superficial stains or defects. Since that time, Croll further modified the technique, reducing the concentration of the acid to approximately 11% and increasing the abrasiveness of the paste using silicon carbide particles (in a water-soluble gel paste) instead of pumice which is marketed as Prema compound (Premier Dental Products Co., Plymouth Meeting, PA) or Opalustre (Ultradent Products, Inc., South Jordan, UT), represents an improved and safer means for the removal of superficial stains or defects. This technique involves the physical removal of tooth structure and does not remove stains or defects through any bleaching phenomena. In 1989, Kamp reported the use of 35% phosphoric acid instead of hydrochloric acid and was considered advantageous as it is commercially used in clinical practice for other procedures.

Advantages:

- Safe and conservative treatment
- Minimal loss of enamel
- Leaves enamel surface lustrous and shiny
- Inexpensive.
- Fast acting.
- Removes yellow-brown, white, and multi-coloured stains.
- Lasting stable aesthetic results
- Results are permanent.

Disadvantages:

- It removes enamel.
- Hydrochloric acid compounds are caustic.
- It requires protective apparatus for patient, dentist, and assistant.

Mechanism of Action

The substance can erode and abrade the enamel surface while removing the stain when applied in a rotational motion. An amorphous, prism-less layer is formed by reshaping the enamel surface layer; this layer is smooth and glossy to the naked eye. This effect has been called "Enamel Glaze" or "Abrasion Effect".

Procedure

1. Clinical evaluation of the teeth:
   - Before and after the micro abrasion method evaluation, the teeth should be in their normal moist condition, completely covered in saliva.
   - If, following a bleaching treatment, white spots are still visible on the enamel, micro abrasion can be employed to either completely eradicate or significantly diminish the size of such spots. The effectiveness of the camouflage should be thoroughly assessed before treating any white spots that are clearly visible.
2. Equipment needed:
   - Contra angle slow hand piece
   - Micro abrasion material
   - Polishing a prophylaxis paste
   - Rubber cup
3. Patient protection: Gingival protection is normally required
   - Clean teeth with rubber cup & prophylaxis paste
   - Isolate the teeth: rubber dam is best method, with light-cured resin applied to gingiva. The rubber dam can be sealed with copal varnish. Ligature can be tied around the rubber dam.
   - Protect the lips with a Vaseline barrier.
   - Protect soft tissues
4. Miro abrasion reduces the lesion to begin the treatment by using a fine grit diamond on tungsten carbide bur
5. Apply the micro-abrasion compounds to the areas with 60 second interval with appropriate rinsing.
6. Apply the material for short periods of the time only.

7. Caution: If the substance is left for an extended period of time, it might cause harm to soft tissues. This might cause minor ulcers of the mucosa or whiten the gums or other soft tissues.
8. Wipe off first to prevent splashing and washing the teeth.
9. Check periodically from the labio-lingual aspect for the minimal enamel reduction.
10. Repeat the procedure
11. Polish the teeth using fine grit fluoridated prophylaxis paste
12. Rinse the teeth
13. Re-evaluate the teeth when wet as some white areas disappears when teeth become wet
14. Remove rubber dam
15. Apply a topical fluoride gel (neutral sodium fluoride gel) application to the teeth for 4minutes
16. Re-evaluate the result
17. Review the patient 4-6 weeks later

Micro Abrasion and Home Bleaching

It is possible to reevaluate the teeth six weeks after the micro abrasion procedure to see if additional treatment is necessary. If the patient wants to try bleaching at home, we may take impressions, make bleaching trays, and teach them how to utilize them. After micro abrasion, you can get great results with home bleaching.

CHAPTER 11

LASER ASSISTED BLEACHING

DR. SARITA SINGH

Light-Amplification-Stimulated Emission of Radiation, or LASER for short, is a technology innovation.

In order to create a coherent beam of light that is nearly parallel and monochromatic, a laser must excite atoms in a controlled manner so that they emit their energy in phase with one another.

In 1996, the FDA authorized the use of the ION LASER TECHNOLOGY argon and carbon dioxide laser, marking the formal beginning of laser bleaching. In an effort to speed up and improve the bleaching process, a new technology called power bleaching with laser has been devised. Unfortunately, tooth whitening with lasers has been a slow-moving process due to a lack of clinical studies and the expensive cost compared to other light technologies.

Emission of high-power radiation that hits a substrate material in one of three ways—transmission, reflection, or absorption—is the basis of this method; absorption yields the best results. Water, or tissues that contain water, absorb the energy of the CO2 laser very quickly. Tissues with a darker pigmentation absorb the argon laser energy more efficiently.

The bleaching gel is activated by the laser light, which dissociates the oxygen molecules within. This allows the gel to penetrate the enamel layer and remove the stain. In order to shorten the bleaching process, laser assisted bleaching makes use of a laser beam to speed up the release of free radicals within the bleaching gel.

The advantages of the use of laser in teeth bleaching are:

- Increases the speed of the procedure,
- comfort of the patient
- minimal to none after treatment discomfort that are often encountered in light activated teeth bleaching with incoherent light sources.

The disadvantages of the use of laser in teeth bleaching are:

- laser beam could harm the patient or operator by direct beam or reflected light, causing retinal burns
- laser is more expensive
- need qualified personal

Factors such as the laser's power density, the wavelength of the radiant energy it emits, and the beam's temporal characteristics (such as continuous vs. pulsed delivery, pulse rate, and pulse duration) are crucial in determining the target's reaction to laser light.

Types of lasers

Different types of lasers are:

1) Carbon dioxide
2) Argon
3) Diode
4) Neodymium: yttrium-aluminium-garnet (Nd: YAG)
5) Erbium-chromium: yttrium-scandium-gallium-garnet (ErCr: YSGG) Lasers

CO2 laser (10,600 nm)

Invisible infrared light is emitted by a carbon-dioxide laser. The molecules may be precisely targeted by these lasers, and they can quickly break down hydrogen peroxide into oxygen and water by utilizing a catalyst. The catalyst/peroxide combination may be damaging; therefore, exposed soft tissues, eyes, and clothing should be protected.

However, another worry with lasers is the potential for harmful consequences linked to elevated pulpal temperatures in teeth. Using a CO2 laser to bleach teeth raised temperatures by 13.1 to 22.30C with gel on the enamel surface and 6.9 to 16.60C on the pulpal side of the dentine, according to research by Luk et al. The absence of well-designed clinical trials meant that the ADA did not approve this wavelength.

Argon laser (488-514nm)

Although the high expense is a major drawback, an argon laser's visible blue light with high-energy photons effectively stimulates the hydrogen peroxide molecule without the heat side effect. It is a different kind of light that can bleach teeth and photopolymerize resin-based objects. The polymerization reaction's initiator, camphorquinone, has an absorption peak at a wavelength that the argon laser produces wavelength-specific laser lines at.

Diode lasers of 830 and 980 nm wavelengths can be used for tooth bleaching in combination with 35– 50% hydrogen peroxide gel.

The so-called "low-level laser" or "diode laser" works by converting electrical energy into laser energy via a solid arsenate semiconductor, which is often linked to indium, gallium, and aluminium. Because diodes are absorbed by hard tissues and do not emit heat, as well as being manageably sized, their wavelength is well-suited for pigmented tissue absorption. A highly concentrated hydrogen peroxide gel may have a cytotoxic impact, although low intensity laser irradiation may counteract this. This is a crucial concern.

To make the gel, the liquid hydrogen peroxide is combined with a powder that mostly consists of fumed silica and a blue dye. The blue dye is able to manage the controlled breakdown of hydrogen peroxide to oxidizing perhydroxyl free radicals by absorbing the laser wavelength and heating it up. Selective diode laser irradiation with 38% hydrogen peroxide can minimize the period of bleaching without surface change of the enamel, according to research by Dostolova et al. (2004) on removed human maxillary central incisors. A variety of different bleaching lights, including a diode laser, were investigated by Sulieman et al. who found that these lights did not increase the intrapulpal temperature above the critical 5.50C as long as they were used.

Nd: YAG laser

The highest temperature elevation in the pulp was registered with the Nd: YAG laser irrespective of the coloured bleaching gel.

According to a study by Kinoshita et al. (2009), a potassium titanyl phosphate (KTP) laser has been used to remove tetracycline stains from teeth. Neodymium: yttrium-aluminium-garnet (Nd: YAG) lasers are various, and one of them is the KTP laser. Because its 1064 nm laser beam passes through the solid medium of KTP crystal, it appears to be suitable for whitening teeth discoloured with tetracycline. in that point, its wavelength is 532 nm, which is just half of what it was in the beginning. So, KTP is comparable to Nd: YAG in many ways and has certain distinct qualities of its own. While water and hydroxyapatite absorb KTP's green visible light, haemoglobin and melanin do not. Dentin is more easily penetrated by KTP. Because of the lower temperature and greater photon energy, it is appropriate for whitening without harming the pulp tissue, and the temperature does not rise greatly during the process. The chemical and photodynamic processes are facilitated by its very energetic photons, which do not harm either the hard or pulp tissues. Evidence suggests that the KTP laser can outperform LED and diode lasers in terms of effect.

Er: YAG laser

In a study by Kivanc et al temperature increase in the pulp was neglectable. A very low temperature rise of 1.860C was registered by Sari et al.

Laser whitening of the tooth enamel and dentin with neodymium: yttrium-aluminium garnet (Nd: YAG) or erbium: yttrium-aluminumgarnet garnet (Er: YAG) can reportedly restore lost bond strength. But it can be costly and take a long time to implement the agents or processes that were proposed.

Influence of laser on the characteristics and material properties of the teeth

Bleaching a tooth should be done in a way that does not alter its structure or composition in any way. On the other hand, some people had enamel-related negative effects following power bleaching.

Morphological analysis: Dominguez et al. found no notable changes in the surface morphology of the enamel following laser bleaching using diode, KTP, Nd: YAG, and Er: YAG.

Mineral content: Parreiras SO et al (2014) demonstrated a reduction in mineral content following bleaching treatments with 35% HP-based bleaching chemicals, both with and without light activation. For two of the three brands, using a light-activated bleach gel in conjunction with a laser or LED (470 nm/810-830 nm) led to calcium loss that was similar to that of the non-light-activated gel. There was no discernible loss of calcium when the Pola Office (Southern Dental Industries, Sao Paulo, SP, Brazil) was exposed to the LED/laser. No significant differences in levels of calcium and phosphorous was seen after 470/830nm LED/laser bleaching.

Bleaching bovine teeth with a low power diode laser (700 nm) without irradiation significantly reduced enamel crystallinity, according to research. On the other hand, crystallinity rose in tandem with the duration of laser irradiation. The results showed that compared to the bleaching treatment without laser irradiation, the professional bleaching treatment with HP and a diode laser not only had a better bleaching impact, but it also protected the enamel structure from modification.

Caries susceptibility of bleached enamel: In office bleaching with a LED/ Laser (470-790nm) doesn't result in a high susceptibility for caries lesion.

Enamel permeability: Higher permeability of the enamel surface after bleaching procedure with a LED/laser (470- 790nm) and QTH light as compared to the control (35% HP) was reported. There was no significant difference between the two-bleaching protocol.

Bleaching with a 470/830nm LED/laser did not show any statistical difference with baseline with regard to dye penetration.

Camargo SEA et al (2009) measured the depth to which 35% hydrogen peroxide triggered by a Nd: YAG laser or a light-emitting diode (LED) penetrated the pulp chamber of teeth bleached in-office on bovines. They found that activating the bleaching chemical with a Nd: YAG laser or LED boosted its penetration into the pulp chamber.

Chang NYN et al (2017) investigated the effects of laser irradiation and topical fluoride on the morphology, permeability, reflectivity, and acid resistance of dentin and enamel in order to better understand the interaction process and create therapies that work. The findings demonstrated that various laser treatments had a significant impact on the morphology and permeability of the enamel and dentin surfaces. Dentin and enamel surfaces became noticeably rougher and more permeable after exposure to Er: YAG irradiation.

Microhardness: The microhardness test is a suitable test for determining small change in surface that demonstrated the effect of bleaching products on enamel

Zhang et al found no significant changes between the control group and the experimental groups using KTP, diode (980 nm), and blue LED composite curing light (470 nm). Microhardness was unaffected by irradiating the 35% HP gel with or without ACP using a diode laser (830 nm).

Bleaching with an LED/laser (470/830nm, light intensity 200mW, 1 minute laser activation of the gel followed by 2 minutes rest: this process was recorded three times) reduced microhardness, which returned to baseline after immersing in artificial saliva for one week.

Kumar P et al (2016) evaluated and compared the surface microhardness and surface morphology of permanent tooth enamel after ErCr: YSGG laser irradiation and Fluoride application. They concluded that ErCr: YSGG laser irradiation alone or in combination with fluoride gel increases the microhardness of the enamel surface.

Nematianaraki S et al (2015)116 assessed the effect on enamel microhardness of two distinct bleaching methods: plasma arc and GaAlAs laser. Although the reduction was significantly smaller with the plasma arc bleaching method compared to the GaAlAs laser, the results demonstrated that both methods reduced enamel micro-hardness.

Procedure

1) Isolate soft tissue and gingivae.
2) Laser bleaching gel is mixed according to manufacturer's instructions.
3) The gel is placed at a thickness of 1-2 mm on to the buccal surface of the teeth to be bleached.
4) Argon laser light is applied for 30 second about 1-2mm from the buccal surface of each tooth.
5) Laser light at 488nm is applied slowly for 30 seconds and moved from right to left surface.
6) After laser activation gel is left onto tooth surface for another 30seconds.
7) The gel is removed from the surface first by wiping it off and then thoroughly washing as 35% hydrogen peroxide is very causative and can cause soft tissue burns.
8) Gel is reapplied in same manner and for same duration for 5 more times in single visit.
9) Treatment time range from 1-3 hours depending on the treatment protocol.

CHAPTER 12

EFFECTS OF BLEACHING ON RESTORATIONS

DR. DAKSHITA JOY SINHA

Numerous studies have reported that tooth bleaching may adversely affect physical and/or chemical properties of restorative materials.

Effects of dental bleaching on composite resin restorations

- Effect on Surface properties and microhardness

Most studies addressing the effects of bleaching agents on the surface properties of composite showed that the effect of bleaching on the surface texture is material- and time-dependent. Surface roughness and the quantity of porosities in micro filled and hybrid composite resins may be slightly but statistically significantly increased when treated with 10- 16% carbamide peroxide bleaching gels, according to certain scanning electron microscopy (SEM) investigations and profilometric assessments. One scanning electron microscopy (SEM) investigation found that 6% hydrogen peroxide gel applied to a hybrid composite and then periodically stored in saliva might change or reduce the impact of the peroxide by creating a surface-protective salivary layer on the restorative material. Furthermore, microfilled specimens showed cracking following four weeks of treatment with 10% carbamide peroxide. Another objective was to examine the effects of various bleaching techniques on the surface texture of nanocomposites and micro hybrid composites. Surface roughness change was found to be material and time dependant, according to the results. The influence of low concentrations (10-16% concentration) of carbamide peroxide gels on the surface microhardness of restorative composite materials is a matter of debate with regard to the bleaching effect on composites' microhardness. Some studies found that using bleaching gels at home caused composite resins to weaken. Other investigations revealed no significant changes in hardness or even an increase in surface hardness due to the application of at-home bleaching gels. Composites were found to remain rigid and have sufficient tensile strength when treated with in-office teeth whiteners with 35% carbamide peroxide or 35% hydrogen peroxide. Using the Knoop hardness test, Hannig et al. (2007) bleached composite resins showed a considerable reduction in surface hardness, both on the outside and inside of the filler materials. The high levels of oxidation and deterioration in the resinous matrix of the composites were the cause of these outcomes. Researchers Taher NM. et al. found that packable composite resin's surface roughness may be altered after three weeks of being treated with 10% CP. On the other hand, surface microhardness was unaltered. Another investigation indicated that after 28 days of treatment with 15% CP, the surface microhardness and texture of both nanohybrid and packable composite resins did not change.

- Effect on Colour change

For standardized and reproducible evaluation of colour changes of restorative materials, colorimeters are used for analysis of L*a*b* values according to the CIELAB system. Using a spectrophotometer, Li et al (2009) discovered that bleaching nanohybrid and packable composite resins with 15% carbamide peroxide significantly altered their colour. According to Hubbezoglu et al., this variation became more apparent when low-density resins, such microfilled composite resin, were treated with a high peroxide concentration of 35%. They reasoned that the amount of resin matrices and the type of filler were responsible for these outcomes. It has been suggested that the colour instability of restorative materials over time is caused by the oxidation of surface pigments and amine compounds, which is also the usual culprit for changes in the colour of these materials. Varying degrees of resin matrix conversion and resin concentration may account for observed variations in colour shift between materials. Chemically cured composites showed more colour change than light-cured ones for the reasons given above; this discrepancy is mostly due to the activator system's role in the matrix phase's composition. Fay et al. (1999) found that bleaching can remove stains from the external surface of a composite restoration and another study by Turkun and Turkun (2004) found that polishing was less efficient than bleaching with 10-15% hydrogen peroxide in restoring the original colour of the composite resin and eliminating stains. It is recommended to polish restorations after bleaching, at the very least, because some microorganisms that cause cavities are believed to adhere more readily to tooth-coloured restorations after coming into contact with bleaching agents due to the increased surface roughness, as assessed by Mor et al. (1998).

- Effects on marginal quality and microleakage

A study by Crim et al (1992) assessed how bleaching excised teeth affected the microleakage of Class V composite resin restorations that were later installed. As a control, ten removed premolars were kept in irater at 37°C. Ten primary teeth were left in a carbamide peroxide gel for nine days, with each session lasting two hours. Outside of treatment times, these samples were kept in water at 37 degrees Celsius. The cementoenamel junction on the lingual and facial surfaces of each tooth was subsequently prepared for a Class V cavity. Each group had half of their teeth repaired using Prisma Universal Bond 3/AP.H. and half with Scotchbond 2/Silux Plus. After being immersed in water at 370°C for 24 hours, the teeth underwent 100 cycles of thermal stress. Dye penetration was used to measure microleakage. This study's findings proved that whitening teeth before dental restorations had no effect on the marginal seal of the final restorations. Microleakage rates of labial restorations with enamel borders only were shown to be considerably elevated following 10% carbamide peroxide bleaching, according to another study by Ulukapi et al. (2003). In contrast, another study by White et al (2008) discovered no elevated rates of microleakage, particularly along the edges of the enamel. The researchers in that study discovered that using 20% carbamide peroxide to bleach teeth with Class I composite restorations did not lead to microleakage since it did not impact the restorations' occlusal margins. Ajami et al. (2012) Researchers found that using mouthrinses like Oral-B after bleaching can make resin composite restorations bonded using etch-and-rinse adhesive systems more susceptible to microleakage after the restoration.

- Effects on the bonding of composite resin restorations to tooth structure

You may classify the effects of dental bleaching on the bonding capacity of composite resin restorations to tooth structure into two categories: those that occur before the operation and those that occur after the procedure. Dental bleaching's effect on adhesive restorations' ability to attach to tooth structure has been the subject of much research. Some writers have postulated that any remaining peroxide on the tooth's surface weakens the connection because it gets in the way of resin bonding and stops it from being fully polymerized. Some have hypothesized that diminished bond strength could be the result of essential bleaching changing the protein and mineral composition of the enamel's outer layers. A variety of approaches have been put forth in the literature to strengthen the connection of teeth that have been bleached before. Research has shown that 10% sodium ascorbate can restore the bond strength of resin composites that were previously bonded to enamel that had been bleached with 10% carbamide peroxide. Lai et al. (2002) discovered that the bond strength of teeth bleached with sodium hypochlorite or hydrogen peroxide may be instantly restored with a surface treatment of an antioxidant (sodium ascorbate). Moreover, in a study conducted by Feiz et al. (2011), Composite resin bond strength to bleached dentin might be enhanced by adding sodium ascorbate, an antioxidant, to the mix. However, adding calcium hydroxide, a buffering agent, had no effect on bond strength. Sodium ascorbate hydrogel application following bleaching increased the resin-enamel bond strength, and this was directly proportional to its duration of application, according to another study by Dabas et al. (2011). The study tested the effects of 10% and 20% hydrogel on the bond strength of bleached enamel for 30, 60, and 120 minutes. Even when the concentration of sodium ascorbate hydrogel was increased, the bond strength remained same. Furthermore, Danesh-Sani and Esmaili (2011) proved that putting off the bonding process until one week after bleaching decreased the composite resin's impaired SBS and polymer made of glass and resin. Additionally, when restoration can be done right after bleaching, using 10% sodium ascorbate hydrogel to treat bleached enamel surfaces restored the weakened SBS and might be a substitute for delayed bonding. Furthermore, other research has shown that the effectiveness of antioxidants as reducing agents can be influenced by the adhesives' chemical makeup and the way they are applied. Khoroushi and Saneie (2012) performed three sets of experiments on bleached enamel: just after bleaching, after a one-week delay, and after applying an antioxidizing agent. The goals were to compare the SBS of three distinct adhesive procedures: three-step etch & rinse, two-step etch & rinse, and one-step self-etch. There was a statistically significant difference between the unbleached control group and the sodium ascorbate group for three-step etch & rinse, but no difference for two-step etch & rinse. On the other hand, for one-step self-etch, the sodium ascorbate group had a substantially lower shear bond strength (SBS) than the unbleached control group. Sung et al. (1999) offered the use of organic solvent-containing dental adhesives as a means to improve bond strength. When restorative treatment is to be completed right after bleaching (10% carbamide peroxide, Nite White Whitening System), they suggested using an alcohol-based bonding agent (OptiBond) to ensure composite bond strength is not compromised. However, Montalvan et al. (2006) found no difference in SBS between acetone- or ethanol-based adhesives 24 hours after bleaching with 35% hydrogen peroxide (Opalescence Xtra, Ultradent). On the contrary, Niat et al. (2012) indicated that the acetone-based adhesive (One Step) had a higher bond strength than did the alcohol-based adhesive (Single Bond). The binding strength of bleached enamel is significantly increased when a-tocopherol is formulated in solution, according to some research.134 However, they mentioned that a period of at least 1 week after the bleaching treatment is still recommended before bonding procedures can precede. In addition, Vidhya et al. (2011) found that oligomeric proanthocyanidin complexes (OPCs) derived from grape seed extract, when applied to enamel before bonding processes and after 38% hydrogen peroxide bleaching, entirely mitigate the bleaching's negative effects and considerably enhance bond strength. The literature suggests that the best course of action is to delay the bonding procedure for a certain amount of time following tooth bleaching, which can range from 24 hours to one week, two weeks, or even four weeks, since the decrease in bond strength following dental bleaching can be reversed.

Multiple approaches were employed to investigate the bonding potential effect of post-operative tooth whitening. These methods included measuring bond strength, fracture toughness, and microleakage. Peroxide bleaching products create oxygen radicals, which are known to be very reactive and nonspecific. These radicals might potentially harm teeth tissues, restorative materials, and the bond between them are all susceptible to degradation to varying degrees. Tissues and restorative materials can impact tooth chemical structure through reductions in the Ca/P ratio, enamel microhardness, dentin permeability, and surface morphology, while surface microhardness, colour changes, surface properties, and marginal integrity can impact restorative materials.

Cavalli et al. (2005) bonded composite-tooth interfaces with two adhesive systems—Single Bond (SB) and Clearfil SE Bond (CB)—to enamel and dentin, and then applied a bleaching chemical comprising 10% carbamide peroxide. Bleaching had a notable effect on CB binding strength to enamel, but had no effect on dentin bond strength for either adhesive method, according to the results. Bleaching may also reduce the interfacial fracture toughness of dentin-resin composite adhesive surfaces, according to Far and Ruse (2003). Barcellos et al. (2010) evaluated the effect of bleaching gel containing 10%, 15%, and 20% carbamide peroxide on the bond strength of dental enamel or dentin and resin composite restorations. Results showed that carbamide peroxide bleaching agents could significantly affect the micro-tensile bond strength (micro-TBS) between the restoration and dental structure. Moreover, they determined that the restoration-dental structure bond strength is worsened by an increase in carbamide peroxide concentration, and that the bond to dentin of the resin composite was less affected by this negative effect compared to the bond to the enamel substrate. Research on the impact of over-the-counter bleaching agents on dental restorations has also shown conflicting findings. Using a home whitening gel for four weeks to treat a hybrid resin composite considerably lowered its hardness, according to one study. Surface cracking was also seen by scanning electron photomicrographs. Glass ionomers show the most noticeable change in colour when exposed to whitening chemicals, however this is not the case for all restorative materials. Porcelain, resin composite, amalgam, or gold restorations were not negatively affected in either surface texture or colour by whitening treatments, according to another study. The pH of whitening chemicals may be linked to their ability to negatively impact restorative materials, according to some studies. This is because treatments with pH values below 5.5 have been found to have more significant impacts.

- Effects of dental bleaching on Amalgam and other dental alloys

Dental amalgams treated to carbamide peroxide solutions for durations varying from 8 hours to 14 to 28 days exhibited an increase in mercury release, according to the studies. From four to thirty times more than in saline controls, the amount of mercury emitted varied with amalgam type and bleaching chemical type. There is a direct relationship between the concentration of peroxide and the amount of mercury released. The older the dental amalgam, the rougher its surface, and the more acidic the bleaching solution, the more mercury is released. Amalgam is thought to emit more mercury than other dental fillings because of the bleaching chemicals' oxidizing effects. To lessen the likelihood of corrosion, it is recommended to polish amalgam restorations before beginning bleaching treatment. This will decrease the amount of time patients spend in contact with amalgam components. Additionally, pre- coating of amalgam surfaces with a protective varnish such as copalite (10% copal resin in a combination of ether, alcohol and acetone) seems to be advisable to reduce release of mercury into the surrounding environment during bleaching with 10% carbamide peroxide. Dental amalgams treated with 10% CP did not exhibit a notable rise in the release of metal ions, according to Al-Salehi and colleagues. In contrast, research has shown that dental amalgams subjected to concentrations of 10% CP or 1%, 3%, 10%, or 30% HP release metal ions at a significantly higher rate. Differences in peroxide concentration and application duration may be at the root of this debate.

A number of studies have found that CP and HP change the properties of dental amalgam restorations, such as colour, marginal adaptability, elution, microhardness and surface roughness.

- Effect of colour changes and marginal adaptability

A patient who underwent a lengthy bleaching procedure with 10% CP developed a green discoloration surrounding certain dental amalgam restorations, according to a case report written by Haywood. Dental amalgam removal exposed carious lesions beneath the surface. No degradation was discovered when other amalgam restorations that did not exhibit greening were removed from the same patient. That being the case, the discolouration may have its roots in the amalgam restoration's little imperfections. Before bleaching, dentists should carefully inspect the restorations for greening discolouration; pay special attention to the amalgams with minor inconsistencies In a different case study, the bleaching tray became stained in spots where dental amalgam restorations showed signs of superficial chipping at the cavosurface borders, which occurred after intraoral bleaching with 10% CP. Possible reasons for the observed colour shift in these case reports include bleaching agent and dental amalgam composition, untreated decay, flawed amalgam restorations, or a combination of these factors.

- Effect on surface properties

Neither type III gold alloy nor high- copper amalgam undergoes surface texture changes when exposed to low-concentration hydrogen peroxide gels (6%). Corrosion of non-polished amalgam samples and nickel-chromium specimens may occur when a 10% carbamide peroxide solution is applied to these materials, according to corrosion current density evaluations of several dental alloys; however, noble metals were not affected. Another study found that using 10% and 35% CP for 14 days, respectively, to mimic at-home and in-office bleaching, altered the surface topography of gold, NieCr, and CoeCr alloys.

- Effect on Surface microhardness

Results from scanning electron microscopy analysis of surfaces treated with HP bleaching on gold alloys did not indicate any major adverse effects. Research has shown that whitening toothpaste containing peroxide affects surface roughness and microhardness of commercially pure titanium and titanium-tantalum alloys differently than toothpaste without peroxide. This contradicts the research that found no modification of gold alloys. Having said that, there was no statistically significant bleaching impact. In general, the investigations showed that bleaching dental amalgam restorations had small, manageable impacts on elution, surface roughness, and microhardness.

- Effects of dental bleaching on Dental ceramic

Although conventional dental ceramics are considered the most inert among dental restorative materials, feldspathic porcelain exhibited surface deterioration in contact with 10% and 35% CP for 21 days.

- Effect on surface roughness

After highly concentrated HP application (30%, 35%, 38%), the surface roughness of alumina-reinforced dental ceramic increased significantly with time of immersion as well as with the increase in concentration of HP.

- Effect on microhardness

Thirty days following bleaching with 10% and 16% CP, Turker and Biskin discovered that the surface microhardness of feldspathic porcelain decreased by a substantial 15%. Schemehorn et al. also observed in their scanning electron microscopy (SEM) study that using a 6% hydrogen peroxide gel on feldspathic porcelain had no effect on surface roughness. Another study by Zaki and Fahmy categorize ceramic repairs as either autoglazed or overglazed. Polished overglazed ceramic restorations had their surface roughness and whiteness altered by an in-office bleaching process using 35% CP followed by an at-home bleaching method using 15% CP; autoglazed restorations were unaffected. Reason being, higher plaque retention, bacterial adhesion, and gingival irritation may result from the rougher ceramic. Malkondu et al (2011) reported that 35% CP induced a reduction in surface microhardness of both leucite reinforced and conventional glass ceramic. Overall, these studies show that bleaching could affect the microhardness and surface roughness of porcelain.

- Effects of dental bleaching on Glass Ionomer Cement and Resin-Modified Glass Ionomer Cement

Some studies have evaluated the effects of bleaching agents on glass ionomer and resin modified glass ionomer cements.

- Effect on colour

A recent in situ study by Li and colleagues (2009) found a significant difference in the colour of a conventional glass ionomer cement restoration after 4 weeks of bleaching with 15% CP. However, 2 weeks after the whitening treatment ceased, the colour returned to that noted before the treatment, showing that bleaching did not affect the colour of the glass ionomer cement.

- Effect on the surface properties and microhardness

Scanning electron microscopy (SEM) revealed a slight surface dissolution. Another research came to a similar conclusion, explaining surface changes like cracks and pits in the glass ionomer cement as a result of the bleaching agent's capacity to change the material's surface characteristics. They also discovered that several staining solutions, including red wine, herbal tea, Coca-Cola, and coffee, had a pH ranging from 3.73 to 6.25 and were more likely to damage bleached glass ionomer restorations. The surface hardness and softening impact of resin modified glass ionomer cement restorations were observed to be significantly reduced when 15% CP and 35% HP were applied, according to Taher NM et al. (2005). After at-home bleaching with 15% CP, there was a 2.6% increase in hardness compared to the control group. The percentage decrease for in-office bleaching with 35% HP was 23.1%. Multiple air bubbles incorporated with the material, which might alter the final qualities of the restorations, was the reason they ascribed these outcomes to. Bleaching changes glass ionomer and resin-modified glass ionomer cement restorations, therefore it may be necessary to replace them. Surface microhardness was either enhanced or maintained following 10% CP treatment with resin-modified glass ionomer cement. One theory put the increased surface microhardness of resin-modified glass ionomer cement's bleaching agent erosion at the root of the problem. A notable reduction in the surface microhardness of resin-modified glass ionomer cement was noted when a more intense bleaching regime of 15% CP and 35% HP was used.

- Effects of dental bleaching on Compomer (Polyacid-Modified Composite Resin)

The addition of fluoroaluminosilicate glass to composite resins gives them characteristics comparable to glass ionomers, including the ability to release fluoride. Bleaching changes the colour, texture, and hardness of a material, according to studies.

- Effect of bleaching on the roughness

Research in humans has demonstrated that bleaching processes considerably raise the surface roughness of compomers. Following treatment with 10% and 15% CP, scanning electron microscopy revealed surface dissolving, fractures, and chemical changes in the restorations. One study related these results to filler matrix debonding at the surface of the compomer, caused by free radicals from the peroxide.

- Effect of bleaching on the colour

Li Q et al (2009) and Yu H et al (2009) assessed the impact of bleaching on the colour of composite restorations and found that using 10% to 15% CP bleaches produces a noticeable shift, which may be associated with changes to the surface. Yu H et al (2009) found that following bleaching with 15% CP, composite restorations were more likely to become stained by red wine, coffee, and Coca-Cola.

- Effect of bleaching on the hardness

Bleaching agents were previously found to soften the subsurface layers of compomer up to 2 mm. The CP-treated composite showed both surface and subsurface changes, including fractures and dissolution, which may explain why the flexural strength decreased and the staining sensitivity increased following bleaching. Rosentritt and colleagues (2005) discovered that bleaching caused the compomers to degrade and lose some of their hardness. Another research found that bleached compomers had a noticeable effect on layers as thick as 2 mm, causing a considerable decrease in hardness and giving the impression that the filler materials had softened. According to Wattanapayungkul et al. (2004), the surface change of the composite was induced by the filler-matrix debonding that occurred as a result of the bleaching agents' oxidation effects. In sum, the results of these investigations demonstrated that bleaching chemicals can have a clinical impact on the microhardness, colour stability, stain susceptibility, and roughness of composite restorations.

- Effects of dental bleaching on Ormocer (Organically Modified Ceramic)

Ormocers, or organically modified ceramics, are a combination of organic and inorganic copolymers developed to improve the results of dental restorations.

- Effect on stability of the colour

Studies investigated the impact of bleaching agents on the stability of the colour of ormocer restorations. Using a colorimeter, Yalcin and Gurgan (2005) found a significant change in the colour of samples of ormocer exposed to 10% CP. Another study that used a high (35%) concentration of HP demonstrated a significant change in colour that could necessitate the replacement of the restoration.

- Effect on microhardness

According to Taher NM.et al (2005), Even when exposed to a highly concentrated peroxide solution, such as 35% HP, the microhardness of ormocers remained somewhat unchanged. They concluded that the ormocers matrix, which includes inorganic-organic copolymers, and the high weight proportion of filler particles were responsible for these outcomes. Two more investigations also found comparable outcomes with doses of 38% HP and 15% CP. Since the ormocers' microhardness did not change, they thought bleaching was a safe alternative that would not need replacing the restorations.

- Effect on the elution of monomers

Polydorou O et al (2008) tested several dental materials for monomer elution after bleaching. After comparing the amounts of bisphenol, A emitted by bleached and unbleached ormocer samples, they determined that bleaching the restorations does not pose a health risk.

- Effects of dental bleaching on Provisional materials

When the access cavity was provisionally restored using temporary restorative materials like TERM, zinc-oxide-eugenol cement, or zinc oxide phosphate cement, the walking-bleach technique, which involves using a bleaching agent mixture of 30% hydrogen peroxide and sodium perborate, failed to produce an optimal seal. When evaluated for a temporary seal of the access cavity, it was equally true for composite materials placed without the acid-etching process. The most favourable results with respect to cavosurface seal during internal bleaching were demonstrated for hydraulic filling materials, such as Cavit and Coltosol. Jefferson et al. (1992) described a decrease in aluminium and an increase in porosity in zinc oxide cement after immersion in acidic 10% carbamide peroxide solutions. Zinc oxide surface levels of IRM fillings were significantly reduced due to influence of 10% carbamide peroxide, but not after application of 10% hydrogen peroxide, which, however, led to cracking and expansion of the tested material. The colour of provisional restorative materials designed for fabrication of crowns were reported to change after 14 days of simulated bleaching with 10% carbamide peroxide gel dependent on the provisional material tested.

- Penetration of the pulp chamber by bleaching agents in restored teeth

It was observed that during external bleaching with 30% hydrogen peroxide or 10–35% carbamide peroxide gel higher levels of hydrogen peroxide penetrated into the pulp chamber in teeth with restorations placed in enamel as compared to sound teeth. This was true for restorations fabricated with either composite materials, polyacid- modified composite resins or resin-modified glass ionomer cements. Furthermore, it was shown that higher concentrated carbamide peroxide gels (35%) lead to distinct higher levels of peroxide in the pulp chamber compared to low (10%) concentrated gels.

CHAPTER 13

ADVERSE EFFECTS OF TOOTH BLEACHING

DR. KASHAF RAZA

The side effects of tooth bleaching can manifest both locally and systemically.

Local Effects on Dental Tissues and Oral Mucosa

The whitening properties of hydrogen peroxide on teeth and the oral mucosa are extensively documented. However, in a small percentage of cases, adverse reactions such as hypersensitivity (ranging from 2.62% to 3.38%) and gingival irritation (between 0.23% and 0.85%) have been observed. Additionally, research has noted alterations in enamel microhardness, the presence of micromorphological defects resulting from demineralization, and its impact on restorative materials.

Cervical root resorption

linked to intracoronal bleaching was first documented by Harrington and Natkin in 1979. This phenomenon, which involves the progressive loss of root structure, remains a significant concern in dental practice. Several factors have been identified as potential contributors to cervical resorption, including trauma, intracoronal bleaching procedures, surgical interventions, orthodontic treatment, periodontal therapy, bruxism, delayed eruption, developmental abnormalities, intracoronal restorations, and advancing age. Among these, the combination of prior dental trauma and bleaching has been highlighted as the most significant risk factor.

Incidence and Prevalence: A study conducted by Heithersay analyzing cases of cervical resorption found that 24.1% were linked to orthodontic treatment, 15.1% to dental trauma, 5.1% to surgical procedures, and 3.9% to intracoronal bleaching.

Mechanism of Resorption: The exact process by which bleaching contributes to cervical resorption remains unclear. One hypothesis suggests that hydrogen peroxide may penetrate dentinal tubules, cementum, and the periodontal ligament, triggering an inflammatory response. This, in turn, could lead to dentin protein denaturation, a reduction in pH, and osteoclastic activation, ultimately resulting in resorption. Lado et al proposed that bleaching agents, through oxidation, induce dentin protein denaturation, prompting a foreign body reaction. It has been further theorized that this denaturation may be driven by exposure to heat or fluctuations in pH caused by bleaching agents.

Impact of Different Techniques and Material Properties on Resorption Bleaching Techniques: Two primary techniques are employed for internal bleaching: the chairside technique and the walking bleach technique.

Chairside Technique: The chairside method utilizes Superoxyl at a concentration of 30– 35%, hydrogen peroxide (H_2O_2), and heat. While this approach is highly effective in whitening, the potent oxidizing agent poses a risk of tissue damage. Studies indicate a 6–8% incidence of cervical resorption, with the risk escalating to 18–25% when heat is applied in conjunction with the bleaching agent. The thermocatalytic approach, which involves heat application, results in an expansion of dentinal tubules, thereby enhancing the diffusion of molecules into the dentin. As temperature increases, the permeability of hydrogen peroxide within the dentin rises, facilitating its deeper penetration. Additionally, heat accelerates the breakdown of hydrogen peroxide into highly reactive hydroxyl radicals, which have been demonstrated to degrade connective tissue components. Consequently, due to the significant risk of external root resorption associated with heat exposure, the thermocatalytic technique has seen reduced clinical use.

Walking Bleach Technique: The walking bleach method involves the application of a mixture of sodium perborate with either water or 30% hydrogen peroxide (Superoxol). Notably, studies have shown that using a sodium perborate–hydrogen peroxide solution does not lead to cervical resorption, even after one year of bleaching. This could be attributed to sodium perborate's ability to suppress macrophage activity. Since macrophages play a pivotal role in stimulating osteoclastic bone resorption and contributing to the degradation of dentin and cementum through lytic processes in periodontal tissues, their inhibition may help prevent resorption. However, despite being considered a safer bleaching agent, sodium perborate has exhibited cytotoxic effects on periodontal ligament cells in in vitro studies, suggesting potential risks with prolonged exposure.

Types of Bleaching Agents: A comparison of different bleaching materials reveals that 35% carbamide peroxide exhibits the lowest levels of extra radicular diffusion, while 35% hydrogen peroxide demonstrates the highest, with sodium perborate falling between the two. Given its minimal diffusion beyond the root structure and proven effectiveness as an intracoronal bleaching agent, 35% carbamide peroxide may be considered the preferred choice for internal bleaching.

This preference is attributed to three key factors:

1. Alkaline pH – Upon breakdown, carbamide peroxide releases ammonia, leading to an alkaline environment within the tooth. This reduces the etching effect on dentin, thereby minimizing structural degradation.
2. Lower Hydrogen Peroxide Yield – The decomposition of carbamide peroxide results in the release of only 12% hydrogen peroxide, significantly less than that of pure hydrogen peroxide- based agents.
3. Slower Diffusion Through Dentin – The gradual diffusion rate allows for greater deionization, reducing the amount of unreacted hydrogen peroxide that reaches the root surface, thereby decreasing the risk of adverse effects.

Due to these properties, carbamide peroxide is often regarded as a safer and more effective option for intracoronal bleaching.

Acidic pH and Its Effects on Dentin: Bleaching agents have been found to induce superficial structural changes in dentin. Their acidic pH enhances dentin permeability by dissolving the smear layer that normally covers the exposed surfaces of dentinal tubules. This increased permeability facilitates the diffusion of hydrogen peroxide through the tubules. If its concentration exceeds a critical threshold, it may contribute to cervical root resorption.

According to Halliwell et al., hydrogen peroxide concentrations below 20 mol/L are considered safe, whereas levels exceeding 50 mol/L exhibit cytotoxic effects on most living cells. A study by Price et al. (2000) examined the pH levels of various bleaching agents and found that most in-office bleaching products were acidic. Since highly concentrated hydrogen peroxide solutions tend to be acidic, they may pose a risk of tissue damage. The acidic environment Favors osteoclastic activity, which can accelerate bone resorption, further emphasizing the need for caution when selecting bleaching agents.

Impact of Cementum Loss on Resorption: When bleaching is performed on teeth with exposed dentinal tubules at the cementoenamel junction (CEJ)—whether due to anatomical defects or cervical erosion—using bleaching agents with high concentrations of active oxidizing compounds should be avoided.

Research by Rotstein et al. indicates that when root cementum is absent, up to 82% of a 30% hydrogen peroxide solution applied within the pulp chamber can diffuse through the root structure. Even when using a sodium perborate-based mixture with hydrogen peroxide or water, complete prevention of peroxide diffusion into dentin is not possible. However, the extent of diffusion is significantly lower when sodium perborate-tetrahydrate mixed with water is used instead of a 30% hydrogen peroxide-sodium perborate combination. Although this technique reduces peroxide penetration into surrounding tissues, a proper cervical seal remains essential. The absence of this seal is another contributing factor that increases the risk of hydrogen peroxide diffusing into periodontal tissues.

Preventive Strategies to Reduce Resorption Risk

1. Use of Protective Barriers

Rotstein and colleagues suggest that placing a protective cement barrier over the gutta-percha, ensuring it does not extend beyond the cervical margin, can effectively limit the diffusion of 30% hydrogen peroxide through radicular dentin. This barrier helps prevent bleaching agents from leaking and infiltrating the spaces between the gutta-percha and the root canal walls, thereby reducing the risk of peroxide reaching the periodontal ligament through dentinal tubules, lateral canals, or the root apex.

2. Avoiding Strong Oxidizers

Since 30% hydrogen peroxide is a key contributor to dentin and cementum degradation, clinicians should consider avoiding its use in internal bleaching to prevent external root resorption. While hydrogen peroxide enhances bleaching efficiency, alternative approaches, such as multiple applications of sodium perborate, provide effective yet safer results. Sodium perborate is a milder bleaching agent that typically does not require additional soft tissue protection.

3. Avoiding Acid Etching

Some clinicians have proposed acid etching as a method to remove the smear layer within the pulp chamber, facilitating better penetration of the bleaching agent. However, this technique increases the permeability of dentin, enhancing peroxide diffusion, which may elevate the risk of resorption.

4. Avoiding Heat Application

Excessive heat during bleaching can cause damage to cementum, periodontal ligament, dentin, and enamel. The risk is particularly high when heat is combined with strong oxidizing agents, making its use in internal bleaching inadvisable.

Treatment Approaches for Cervical Resorption

Various treatment strategies have been proposed over time, with the prognosis depending on the extent of the resorption process. Treatment selection is guided by the severity of the lesion:

1. Conservative Approaches for Early-Stage Resorption
   - Remineralization can be attempted in early-stage resorption by applying calcium hydroxide, which induces an alkaline environment that discourages further osteolytic activity.
   - Friedman et al. recommend calcium hydroxide recalcification treatment to stimulate reparative hard tissue formation, as suggested by Tronstad et al.
   - However, if communication exists between the resorption site and the oral cavity, recalcification treatment may fail, necessitating surgical intervention.

2. Surgical and Restorative Treatments for Advanced Cases

   - Direct Restoration: If cervical resorption is surgically accessible, a direct restoration may be placed. However, this technique has limitations:
     - the affected area may not be entirely instrumented during the procedure, allowing continued resorption.
     - Surgical intervention may compromise periodontal health and aesthetics.
   - Crown Lengthening and Orthodontic Extrusion:
     - If resorption has progressed, a crown lengthening procedure or forced orthodontic eruption may be necessary to expose sound tooth structure before restoring the defect.
     - Inflammatory osteolytic lesions typically have a low pH, which promotes hard tissue resorption. Root canal dressings containing calcium hydroxide can counteract this by raising the pH and reducing further degradation.

- o If the lesion is subgingival or extends below the bone crest, a labial flap may be required to allow proper cleaning and restoration of the defect.
- o Trichloroacetic acid (90%) can be applied to the affected margins to necrotize granulation tissue before placing a suitable restorative material.

3. Complex Cases and Alternative Approaches

- In cases where external root resorption is extensive, a combined endodontic-periodontal approach may be beneficial.
  - o A reported technique involved restoring the coronal portion of the defect with composite resin, while using mineral trioxide aggregate (MTA) for the portion extending below the bone.
  - o However, research suggests that bleaching can increase resin solubility and weaken enamel bond strength, leading to higher marginal leakage.

4. Extraction as a Last Resort

- If external root resorption cannot be controlled, extraction is often the only viable treatment.

Post-Treatment Hypersensitivity and Pulp Alterations

Tooth sensitivity is a common side effect of external tooth bleaching, typically lasting up to four days after treatment cessation. Research indicates that sensitivity peaks around the third day of bleaching, likely due to the maximum saturation of oxygen inside the pulp at that stage.

Mechanism of Tooth Sensitivity:

The exact mechanisms behind tooth sensitivity following bleaching are not fully understood. However, it is believed that hydrogen peroxide (H_2O_2) and free radicals penetrate enamel and dentin, reaching the pulp chamber, where they trigger pulpal inflammation. This inflammation leads to heightened sensitivity, particularly in response to cold stimuli, until the inflammation subsides.

Several theories attempt to explain this sensitivity:

1. Direct Innervation Theory:

    - Suggests that nerve endings penetrate dentin and extend to the dentin-enamel junction (DEJ), causing sensitivity upon mechanical stimulation.
    - However, this theory lacks strong evidence because:
        - Superficial dentin does not contain many nerve fibres.
        - The plexus of Raschkow, responsible for dentinal nerve fibres, does not fully develop until complete tooth eruption.

2. Odontoblast Receptor Theory:

    - Proposes that odontoblasts act as receptors, transmitting signals to nerve endings.
    - This theory has been rejected since the cellular matrix lacks the ability to generate nerve impulses.

3. Hydrodynamic Theory (Most Accepted Theory):

    - States that fluid movement within dentinal tubules, particularly around odontoblasts, excites nerve endings, triggering pain.
    - Bleaching increases permeability, making teeth more susceptible to this effect

On a molecular level, peroxide-induced sensitivity is linked to the activation of TRAP1 (transient receptor potential cation channel with ankyrin domain-type 1). Peroxide oxidizes cysteine residues in TRAP1, and the Fenton reaction (oxidation of Fe^{2+}) plays a role in this activation.

Incidence of Tooth Sensitivity:

Clinical trials estimate that the risk of sensitivity is:

- 51% in at-home bleaching
- 63% in in-office bleaching

At-home bleaching results in lower sensitivity due to the use of lower peroxide concentrations over a longer duration. In-office bleaching, in contrast, involves higher concentrations to compensate for shorter treatment times, increasing sensitivity.

Studies show that:

- 20% hydrogen peroxide in in-office bleaching is as effective as 35% peroxide, but with reduced sensitivity.
- Lower concentrations, such as 6% peroxide, yield less colour change but also less sensitivity.

Bleaching has been successfully used in children and adolescents, but clinicians should closely monitor younger patients due to their newly erupted teeth, which are more permeable and prone to higher sensitivity risks.

Factors affecting sensitivity risk:

- Frequency of daily applications (more frequent applications increase sensitivity).
- Quality of bleaching agents.
- Individual response to treatment.

Interestingly, age, sex, restorations, enamel-cementum abrasion, and dental arch treated do not significantly influence the risk of sensitivity.

Symptoms of Bleaching-Induced Sensitivity:

- Sensitivity is typically mild and transient, occurring early in treatment and subsiding shortly after bleaching ends.
- Patients with a history of sensitivity may be at a higher risk and should be evaluated before treatment begins.
- Clinical studies report

- o Schulte et al. (1994): In a study using 10% carbamide peroxide, 4 out of 28 participants discontinued treatment due to sensitivity, but no significant pulpal changes were noted in others.
- o Sterrett et al. (1995): A three-week study found that all participants experienced mild, transient sensitivity, which disappeared after treatment
- o Kawachi T (1980) & Nathanson D (1997): Two-thirds of patients in trials experienced mild, transient thermal sensitivity, resolving upon bleaching cessation.

Pulp Response and Dentin Adaptation:

- Mild pulpal inflammation may occur, but the irritation is usually minimal.
- Reactionary dentin formation occurs over time, helping reduce hypersensitivity.
- Peritubular dentin formation can lead to a narrowing of dentinal tubules, further decreasing sensitivity.

Management and Treatment of Tooth Sensitivity:

Various strategies help minimize or manage bleaching-induced sensitivity:

Desensitizing Agents

- Potassium Nitrate
  - Reduces nerve excitability by depolarizing nerve endings.
- Sodium Fluoride
  - Strengthens enamel and reduces permeability.
- Calcium Phosphate
- Aids in remineralization, making dentin less permeable.
- Fluoride Varnishes and Adhesives
  - Provide a protective coating to block tubules and minimize sensitivity.

- Pre-Treatment Strategies
  - Fluoride gel or potassium nitrate toothpaste applied 10–30 minutes before whitening.
  - Desensitizing agent application after treatment to mitigate discomfort.
  - Reducing application frequency (e.g., every other day instead of daily).
  - Using potassium nitrate + fluoride toothpaste two weeks before and during bleaching.

Alterations to the Enamel Surface

The effects of bleaching on enamel have been examined in terms of mineral loss, microhardness changes, and surface morphology.

Mineral Loss: Studies indicate that bleaching can lead to mineral depletion; however, natural remineralization mechanisms in the oral environment help counteract these effects. Ruse et al. (1990) observed alterations in the calcium/phosphate ratio in enamel exposed to 35% hydrogen peroxide.

Microhardness Changes: Most scanning electron microscopy (SEM) and microhardness studies report minimal changes to bleached enamel. However, some investigations have documented surface alterations, including depressions, porosity, and erosion.

Surface Morphology Changes: Certain acidic beverages, such as fruit juices, have demonstrated greater demineralization effects on enamel than bleaching agents. A six-month study evaluating 10% carbamide peroxide revealed no adverse effects on enamel morphology. However, some over-the-counter whitening products have been associated with significant enamel damage.

Causes and Prevention: The impact on enamel is largely attributed to the pH of bleaching formulations. Price et al. (2003) analyzed commercially available products and found pH levels ranging from highly acidic to highly basic. Over-the-counter agents tend to be more acidic, leading to increased enamel erosion.

Remineralization from saliva can help restore mineral content, but the organic matrix may be permanently altered. Fluoride-containing bleaching agents have been shown to reduce enamel demineralization and preserve microhardness.

Effects on Dentin

Research has indicated that bleaching can decrease dentin microhardness. Studies by Pecora et al. (1994) and Basting et al. (2003) suggest that both carbamide peroxide and thickening agents contribute to this reduction. Additionally, Tam et al. (2005) found that prolonged exposure weakens dentin's structural integrity.

Bleaching can also affect bonding to enamel and dentin by altering the resin tags and smear layer. Hydrogen peroxide residues may inhibit polymerization, though delaying bonding procedures for two weeks post- bleaching can improve bond strength.

Effects on Oral and Gastric Mucosa

High concentrations of hydrogen peroxide (30-35%) can cause mucosal burns. Animal studies have shown that exposure to as little as 1% H2O2 for 6-48 hours results in epithelial damage and inflammation.

Gingival Irritation: Gingival irritation commonly occurs in tooth bleaching but is generally mild and self-resolving. It is more frequent with ill-fitting trays, high H2O2 concentrations, or gel contact with soft tissues. Protective measures, including proper tray design and gingival barriers, can help minimize irritation

Enzymes such as catalase and peroxidase naturally mitigate hydrogen peroxide toxicity. If tissue burns occur, extensive rinsing, topical anaesthetics, and vitamin E application can aid healing. Sodium bicarbonate can also be used to neutralize chemical burns.

Overall, while bleaching-induced irritation is typically reversible, careful technique and preventive strategies are necessary to minimize risks.

Gastric Mucosal Irritation: Concerns have been raised regarding the accidental ingestion of bleaching gels by patients. Swallowing significant amounts of these substances can lead to toxicity and irritation of both the gastric and respiratory mucosa.

Preventive Measures for Gastric Mucosal Irritation

To minimize the risk of gastric irritation, it is recommended to use a rubber dam during bleaching treatments to prevent the accidental ingestion of the bleaching agent. For at-home bleaching methods prescribed by dentists, patients should take care to avoid overfilling the bleaching trays.

Other Adverse Effects

Additional side effects that have been reported include sore throat, temporomandibular joint dysfunction due to prolonged tray usage, and minor orthodontic tooth movements.

Prevention Strategies

To reduce the likelihood of soft tissue and throat irritation, modifications to the tray or a reduction in application time may be necessary. For temporomandibular discomfort and unintended tooth movement, using a thin tray material (0.40 in) is recommended.

Systemic Effects of Bleaching Agents Allergic Reactions

There have been no documented cases of allergic sensitivity to carbamide peroxide, hydrogen peroxide, or other related peroxo-compounds, though their acute and sub-acute effects are well recognized.

Acute Cytotoxicity

Toxic effects have been observed at doses exceeding 5 g/kg/day in products containing 10% carbamide peroxide. This equates to a hydrogen peroxide intake ranging from 0.3 to 1.8 mg/kg of body weight per day. In animal studies, forced ingestion of 5 to 50 mg/kg of carbamide peroxide resulted in dose-dependent mucosal ulcerations appearing within an hour, though these lesions typically healed within 24 hours. No adverse reactions were noted at doses below 15 mg/kg. Commercially available bleaching gels containing peroxides have been shown to amplify these toxic effects. Acute toxicity cases, including fatalities, have been reported following the ingestion of highly concentrated hydrogen peroxide solutions.

Children under the age of 18 represent the majority of reported cases of hydrogen peroxide poisoning, with ingestion accounting for most exposures. Solutions containing less than 10% hydrogen peroxide generally cause mild irritation, often leading to spontaneous vomiting or slight abdominal bloating. However, exposure to concentrations exceeding 10% can result in severe tissue burns and systemic toxicity. Hydrogen peroxide toxicity is linked to oxidative damage and the formation of gas embolisms, leading to severe physiological consequences. Symptoms of acute hydrogen peroxide poisoning include abdominal and chest pain, difficulty breathing, frothing at the mouth, unconsciousness, sensory and motor impairments, fever, gastric haemorrhage, and liver damage. Though fatalities are rare, they can occur.

Sub-Acute Toxicity

No documented sub-acute effects have been reported in humans. However, in animal studies, toxic effects were observed when daily intake exceeded 30 mg/kg for rats and 26 mg/kg for mice. Hydrogen peroxide concentrations between 0.15% and 0.4% in drinking water led to pathological changes in the stomach, intestines, liver, and kidneys, with higher concentrations (1-2.5%) resulting in fatalities within two to six weeks. Research has also shown that hydrogen peroxide exposure can cause inflammation and impair microcirculation.

Studies have reported that young rats exposed to 1.5% hydrogen peroxide in their drinking water for eight weeks exhibited growth retardation and changes in periodontal tissues. However, clinical data contradicts this, as long-term use of peroxide-based mouth rinses at similar or higher concentrations has been associated with improved periodontal health

Topical application of hydrogen peroxide in humans has been shown to produce hydroxyl radicals, which can trigger lipid peroxidation and DNA damage, leading to cell lysis and death. Certain antioxidants and iron-chelating agents have been found to counteract these effects. The enzyme catalase helps mitigate oxidative damage by breaking down hydrogen peroxide, while vitamin E (α-tocopherol) protects against lipid peroxidation.

Research by Aren G. demonstrated that exposure to 35% carbamide peroxide reduced cell viability to 60% compared to control samples, with this percentage dropping to 43% when exposed to a 20% concentration. The toxic threshold for these bleaching agents is estimated at 50 and 40 μg/ml, respectively. Extrapolating these findings to a 70-kg human suggests that the daily dose should not exceed 10 mg of carbamide peroxide (equivalent to 3.3 mg of hydrogen peroxide) to avoid potential toxicity.

Genotoxicity and Carcinogenic Potential

Genotoxic Effects

Extensive research has been conducted on the genotoxicity of hydrogen peroxide and peroxide-based whitening agents, both in vitro and in vivo, using various biological models, including microbes, plants, insects, cultured mammalian cells, and animals. Li et al. (1996) found that direct exposure to hydrogen peroxide induced genotoxic effects in bacterial cultures and mammalian cells. However, these effects were significantly reduced or eliminated when hydrogen peroxide was metabolized by enzymes such as catalase.

Repeated applications of 30% hydrogen peroxide in the oral cavity have been linked to hyperkeratosis, hyperplasia, and mild dysplasia after 22 weeks, though no malignant tumours were observed. The International Agency for Research on Cancer (IARC) has not found conclusive evidence linking hydrogen peroxide exposure to mutations or cancer in professional settings. However, animal studies have reported the development of duodenal adenomas and carcinomas following prolonged oral administration of hydrogen peroxide.

Carcinogenic Potential: Japanese studies have shown an increased incidence of duodenal adenocarcinoma in mice exposed to a 0.4% hydrogen peroxide solution for up to 100 weeks. Despite these findings, no human cases have been definitively linked to peroxide-induced carcinogenesis.

The IARC has assessed available data and concluded that while there is some evidence of carcinogenicity in animal models, human data remains inconclusive. As a result, hydrogen peroxide is classified as having limited evidence of carcinogenicity in animals and inadequate evidence in humans.

CHAPTER 14

CONCLUSION

DR. KASHAF RAZA

Dental aesthetics, and in particular the colour of teeth, hold considerable significance in contemporary society, as they directly impact an individual's self-esteem, social interactions, and overall quality of life. The perception of a bright, white smile is often associated with health, youthfulness, and social desirability, whereas discoloration or staining of teeth can have profound psychosocial implications. Research has consistently demonstrated that patients with discoloured teeth may experience diminished confidence, reluctance to smile, and self- consciousness in professional and personal settings. Consequently, aesthetic dental treatments aimed at improving tooth colour are increasingly sought after by patients across age groups and demographic profiles.

Tooth coloration is determined by a combination of intrinsic and extrinsic factors. Intrinsic colour refers to the natural hue of the tooth resulting from the optical properties of enamel and dentin, as well as factors affecting the tooth's internal structure. In contrast, extrinsic stains are superficial deposits that accumulate on the tooth surface due to environmental exposures and lifestyle habits. Common contributors to extrinsic discoloration include dietary components such as tannin-rich foods and beverages—most notably red wine, tea, and coffee—as well as smoking and the use of certain medicaments, such as chlorhexidine mouthwashes or metal salts like tin and iron. These external agents interact with the pellicle and enamel surface, causing visible staining that may, over time, penetrate deeper into the enamel and dentin if left untreated. Understanding the aetiology of tooth discoloration is critical for selecting the most appropriate aesthetic intervention, as the nature and depth of the stain influence the choice of treatment and the expected clinical outcome.

A wide array of treatment modalities is available to enhance tooth colour, ranging from minimally invasive approaches to more extensive restorative procedures. Techniques such as microabrasion, veneers, and crowns are employed based on case-specific requirements and patient expectations. Microabrasion is effective in removing superficial enamel defects and discolorations, while veneers and crowns provide a durable solution for teeth with significant intrinsic staining, structural defects, or enamel erosion. Among these, however, tooth bleaching has emerged as one of the most widely utilized contemporary aesthetic procedures, owing to its conservative nature, cost-effectiveness, and ability to safely restore the appearance of both vital and non-vital teeth. Tooth bleaching is generally considered less invasive than restorative alternatives because it does not involve extensive removal of tooth structure, making it the preferred choice for patients seeking non-restorative aesthetic improvements.

Bleaching techniques can be broadly categorized according to the vitality of the teeth. Extra-coronal bleaching refers to the application of bleaching agents externally on the tooth surface, primarily targeting vital teeth with extrinsic stains or mild intrinsic discoloration. In this approach, agents such as hydrogen peroxide or carbamide peroxide are applied via trays, strips, or gels that maintain contact with the tooth surface for a prescribed duration. On the other hand, intracoronal bleaching (also known as internal or non-vital bleaching) is employed for teeth that have undergone endodontic treatment. In these cases, bleaching agents are placed within the pulp chamber, allowing diffusion into dentinal tubules and interaction with chromogenic compounds embedded within the tooth structure. Both approaches aim to modify chromophores in the dentin, resulting in a lighter and more aesthetically pleasing tooth colour. The choice between extra- and intracoronal techniques depends on multiple factors, including tooth vitality, the depth of discoloration, and patient- specific considerations.

The bleaching process is fundamentally dependent on the generation and release of active oxygen species, which diffuse into the dentinal tubules and oxidize the pigmented molecules responsible for discoloration. Most contemporary whitening systems rely on hydrogen peroxide or carbamide peroxide as the primary oxidative agents. Hydrogen peroxide is a powerful oxidant capable of reacting with a wide variety of organic and inorganic substances, effectively breaking down chromophores into smaller, less pigmented fragments. Carbamide peroxide, a compound formed from urea and hydrogen peroxide, serves as a precursor to hydrogen peroxide. When dissolved in water or saliva, carbamide peroxide decomposes into hydrogen peroxide and urea, gradually releasing the active oxidizing species over an extended period. This controlled release allows for safe, prolonged contact with dental tissues, making carbamide peroxide particularly suitable for at-home bleaching protocols. The concentration of bleaching agents, the duration of application, and the mode of delivery are carefully selected to optimize the oxidative effect while minimizing potential adverse outcomes.

Despite their proven efficacy and widespread acceptance, tooth bleaching procedures are not without risks. Among vital teeth, tooth hypersensitivity is the most commonly reported side effect. This transient phenomenon is typically caused by the diffusion of peroxide molecules through enamel and dentin, which can temporarily irritate pulpal nerves. Sensitivity generally manifests as sharp, brief discomfort in response to thermal or tactile stimuli and is often mitigated by reducing application time, lowering peroxide concentration, or using desensitizing agents. In non-vital teeth subjected to internal bleaching, cervical resorption is a recognized complication, arising from the inadvertent penetration of bleaching agents into periapical tissues. Other concerns include potential alterations in enamel microhardness, reduced bond strength of composite restorations, and speculative genotoxic effects. Although the majority of adverse outcomes are temporary and manageable, their existence underscores the importance of careful case selection, adherence to manufacturer protocols, and ongoing professional supervision.

The individualization of bleaching protocols is a critical component in achieving favourable clinical outcomes. Factors such as the type and severity of staining, dietary habits, previous restorative work, and overall oral health must be considered when planning treatment. Teeth with deep intrinsic discoloration may require prolonged or repeated bleaching sessions, whereas extrinsic stains may respond more rapidly to surface-applied agents. Additionally, patients with enamel hypoplasia, cracks, or compromised restorations may necessitate modified protocols to avoid exacerbating existing structural vulnerabilities. The combination of comprehensive diagnostic evaluation, careful treatment planning, and ongoing monitoring ensures that aesthetic objectives are met while preserving tooth integrity.

In clinical practice, bleaching procedures are accompanied by detailed patient education to ensure proper application and to manage expectations regarding the results and potential side effects. Patients are informed about the progressive nature of whitening, the importance of compliance with wear schedules, and the need to avoid foods and beverages that can induce restraining during the treatment period. Follow-up appointments enable the clinician to assess progress, address sensitivity, and adjust the regimen, if necessary, thereby optimizing both the safety and efficacy of the procedure.

Research in tooth bleaching continues to evolve, with ongoing efforts to refine techniques, improve formulations, and reduce adverse effects. Innovations include the incorporation of desensitizing agents, the development of peroxide-free bleaching systems, and the use of light or chemical activators to enhance oxidative reactions. Emerging technologies also focus on improving the diffusion of bleaching agents into dentin while preserving enamel microstructure, allowing for more predictable and durable aesthetic outcomes. The future of bleaching is likely to integrate personalized approaches that consider the patient's unique dental anatomy, stain aetiology, and aesthetic expectations, thereby maximizing both efficacy and satisfaction.

In summary, tooth bleaching is a cornerstone of contemporary aesthetic dentistry, offering a conservative, effective, and patient-centred solution for improving tooth colour. The interplay of intrinsic and extrinsic factors in determining tooth hue necessitates careful diagnosis and individualized treatment planning. Hydrogen peroxide and carbamide peroxide remain the mainstays of bleaching therapy, functioning through the controlled release of oxidative species that interact with chromophores to produce perceptible whitening. While the procedures are generally safe and predictable, attention to potential adverse effects, proper case selection, and ongoing professional supervision are paramount. By integrating scientific understanding with clinical expertise, dental practitioners can restore tooth brightness, enhance patient confidence, and provide durable aesthetic outcomes tailored to each individual's needs.

This book explores the multifaceted aspects of tooth bleaching, including indications, contraindications, techniques, and clinical considerations, providing a comprehensive framework for both research and practice in aesthetic dentistry. The subsequent sections delve into the mechanisms of bleaching, comparative efficacy of different protocols, and the role of patient-centred strategies in achieving optimal results, thereby contributing to the broader understanding of conservative aesthetic interventions in modern dental practice.

BIBLIOGRAPHY

Abuaffan, Amal H. and Mohammed Ibrahim. 2020. "Dental Manifestations in Sickle Cell Anaemia: A Review." *Journal of Clinical and Experimental Dentistry* 12 (5): 411–415.

Alkhatib, Rami, Ruth Holt and Raman Bedi. 2019. "The Relationship Between Oral Hygiene, Plaque Maturation and Pigmented Dental Stains." *Community Dental Health* 36 (1): 43–46.

Alqahtani, Fahad, and Sarah Alquria. 2020. "Color Stability of Restorative Dental Materials: A Contemporary Review." *Journal of Esthetic and Restorative Dentistry* 32 (1): 108–116. DOI: https://doi.org/10.1111/jerd.12530

Alqahtani, Mohammed Q. 2014. "Tooth-bleaching Procedures and Their Controversial Effects: A Literature Review." Saudi Dental Journal 26 (2): 33–46.

Aoba, Toshiaki and Ole Fejerskov. 2019. "Dental Fluorosis: Chemistry and Pathogenesis Revisited." *Caries Research* 53 (2): 190–200.

Attin, T., C. Albrecht, S. Becker, R. Hannig, and R. Wiegand. 2004. "Influence of Carbamide Peroxide on Enamel Surface Properties." Journal of Dentistry 32 (4): 289–294. https://doi.org/10.1016/j.jdent.2004.01.003

Bailey, S. J., and E. J. Swift. 1992. "Effect of Concentration on Carbamide Peroxide Whitening." *Journal of Dentistry* 20 (2): 239–244.

Barcellos, A., et al. 2010. "Effects of Carbamide Peroxide on Bond Strength." *Journal of Esthetic and Restorative Dentistry* 22 (4): 259–266. https://doi.org/10.1111/j.1708-8240.2010.00350.x

Barreto, Ines C., Kelly R. Dos Santos and Alessandro D. Loguercio. 2019. "Extrinsic Tooth Staining: Mechanisms, Prevention and Treatment." *Journal of Esthetic and Restorative Dentistry* 31 (1): 45–52.

Bizhang, M., A. Seemann, T. Duve, A. Römhild, A. Altenburger, and W. W. W. Zimmer. 2006. "In Vitro Evaluation of Tooth Whitening with and without Light Activation." Operative Dentistry 31 (6): 129–135.

Brooks, Cristina, and Michael Reynolds. 2018. "Chemical Mechanisms of Intracoronal Bleaching Agents." Journal of Esthetic and Restorative Dentistry 30 (2): 110–115.

Carey, Clifton M. 2014. "Tooth Whitening: What We Now Know." Journal of Evidence-Based Dental Practice 14: 70–76. https://doi.org/10.1016/j.jebdp.2014.02.006

Carrillo, A., P. Prieto, S. Lusilla, and J. L. Ferrer. 2020. "Clinical Considerations in Tooth Whitening." Journal of Esthetic and Restorative Dentistry 32 (2): 171–178. https://doi.org/10.1111/jerd.12537

Cavalli, Vanessa, Matheus Kury and Priscila B. This. 2022. "Current Status and Future Perspectives of In-Office Tooth Bleaching." *Frontiers in Dental Medicine* 3: 1–8.

Cioni, Ilaria, Andrea Pasqualini, Maria Rossella Baldi, and Giovanni Dolci. 2023. "Evaluation of the Efficacy of Low-Particle-Size Toothpastes against Extrinsic Pigmentations: A Randomized Controlled Clinical Trial." *Dental Journal* 11 (3): 82. https://doi.org/10.3390/dj11030082

Dahl, J. E. 2003. "Tooth Bleaching—A Critical Review of the Biological Aspects." *Critical Reviews in Oral Biology & Medicine* 14 (4): 292-304. https://doi.org/10.1177/154411130301400406

Dahl, J. E., and U. Pallesen. 2003. "Tooth Bleaching—A Critical Review." Journal of the American Dental Association 134 (3): 257–264. https://doi.org/10.14219/jada.archive.2003.0171

De Almeida, L. C. A., et al. 2011. "Effectiveness of Different Application Times of 35% Hydrogen Peroxide." *Journal of Dentistry* 39 (2): 75–82. https://doi.org/10.1016/j.jdent.2010.11.004

de Geus, J. L., A. Wambier, M. Kossatz, A. Loguercio, and A. Reis. 2015. "At-Home Bleaching with Carbamide Peroxide: A Systematic Review and Meta-analysis." Journal of the American Dental Association 146 (2): 262–270. https://doi.org/10.1016/j.adaj.2014.11.012

de Geus, João L., Marcela Ferraz Semensato, Guilherme C. M. Cunha, and Alessandro D. Loguercio. 2020. "Hydrogen Peroxide-Based Whitening: Mechanisms, Sensitivity, and Clinical Considerations." *Journal of Dentistry* 98: 217–224.

de Paula, A. B., et al. 2017. "Tooth Bleaching with Hydrogen Peroxide: A Review." *Brazilian Dental Journal* 28 (2): 112–120. https://doi.org/10.1590/0103-6440201701225

de Paula, A. B., et al. 2017. "Tooth Bleaching with Peroxides: Mechanisms and Effects." *Brazilian Dental Journal* 28 (2): 111–118. https://doi.org/10.1590/0103-6440201701225

Ergin, Osman and Eda Celik. 2019. "Tobacco-Related Tooth Staining and Its Chemical Basis." *Clinical Oral Investigations* 23 (1): 101–105.

Ernani, Vinay and Pavitra Singh. 2021. "Dental Findings in Congenital Erythropoietic Porphyria: A Review." *Oral Diseases* 27 (2): 229–235.

Fasanaro, Anthony M. 1992. "Bleaching Teeth: History, Chemicals, and Methods Used for Common Tooth Discolorations." Journal of Esthetic Dentistry 4 (3): 56–62.
https://doi.org/10.1111/j.1708-8240.1992.tb00876.x

Fioresta, Rossella, María Melo, Leopoldo Forner and José Luis Sanz. 2023. "Prognosis in Home Dental Bleaching: A Systematic Review." *Clinical Oral Investigations* 27 (7): 3347–3361.

Flotra, Liv, Per Gjermo and Gunnar Rolla. 2020. "Chemical Stain Formation Associated with Chlorhexidine Mouthrinses." *Scandinavian Journal of Dental Research* 128 (3): 215–218.

Frank, Ariadne Charis, Philipp Kanzow, Tina Rödig and Annette Wiegand. 2022. "Comparison of the Bleaching Efficacy of Different Agents Used for Internal Bleaching: A Systematic Review and Meta-Analysis." *Journal of Endodontics* 48 (2): 171–178.

Freccia, W. F., and D. D. Peters. 1982. "A Technique for Non-Vital Bleaching: The Thermocatalytic Method." Journal of Endodontics 8 (1): 34–42.

García-Godoy, Franklin and Marie Hicks. 2018. "Bilirubin Staining of Developing Teeth: Clinical and Histological Features." *Pediatric Dentistry* 40 (2): 59–64.

Goldstein, Ronald E., and Daniel A. Garber. 1995. Complete Dental Bleaching. Chicago: Quintessence Publishing.

Gondim, J. O., P. M. Souza, and M. C. Gomes. 2020. "Oxidative Mechanisms in Dental Whitening: Updated Perspectives." Clinical Oral Investigations 24 (1): 209–214.

Greenwall, Linda and Catherine Greenwall-Cohen. 2017. *Tooth Whitening Techniques, 3rd ed.* London: CRC Press. Pages 71–80.

Gür, Gürçağ. 2023. "Non-Vital Discoloured Teeth Bleaching Using the Walking Bleach Technique: A Case Report." *Cumhuriyet Dental Journal* 26 (1): 101–104.

Hasson, Henry J., Amid I. Ismail, and Gregory F. Neiva. 2015. "Home-Based Vital Tooth Bleaching: A Review of Patient-Acceptance Factors." *Operative Dentistry* 40 (1): 79–86.

Haywood, Van B. 2008. "Treating Sensitivity during Whitening." Inside Dentistry 4 (9): 50–56.

Haywood, Van B., and Harold O. Heymann. 1989. "Nightguard Vital Bleaching." Quintessence International 20 (3): 173–176.

Ho, S., M. Goerig, and J. Schaeffer. 1989. "Effectiveness of Sodium Perborate with and without Superoxol in Bleaching of Discoloured Teeth." Journal of Endodontics 15 (5): 255–259.

Jindal, Suman and Harleen Kaur. 2020. "Intrinsic Discoloration of Teeth: Etiology, Diagnosis and Management." *International Journal of Esthetic Dentistry* 15 (2): 88–95.

Joiner, A. 2016. "Tooth Colour: A Review of the Literature." *Journal of Dentistry* 67: 70–83.
https://doi.org/10.1016/j.jdent.2017.09.006

Joiner, A. 2016. "Tooth Whitening: Mechanisms and Safety." *Journal of Dentistry* 67: 70–83.
https://doi.org/10.1016/j.jdent.2017.09.006

Joiner, A., and W. Luo. 2017. "Tooth Colour and Whitening." *Journal of Dentistry* 67: 58–66.
https://doi.org/10.1016/j.jdent.2017.09.006

Joiner, Andrew and Wei-Shao Luo. 2023. "Tooth Colour and Whitening: An Updated Review." *British Dental Journal* 234 (4): 224–229.

Joiner, Andrew, and Wei Luo. 2017. "Tooth Colour and Whitening: An Update on the Latest Evidence." *British Dental Journal* 223 (4): 289–296.

Joiner, Andrew. 2006. "The Bleaching of Teeth: A Review of the Literature." Journal of Dentistry 34 (7): 412–419.
https://doi.org/10.1016/j.jdent.2006.02.002

Joiner, Andrew. 2016. "Tooth Colour: A Review of the Literature." *Journal of Dentistry* 57: 70–84.
DOI: https://doi.org/10.1016/j.jdent.2016.02.002

Justino, L. M., D. R. Tames, and F. F. Demarco. 2004. "In Situ Study of the Effect of Bleaching with Carbamide Peroxide Gel on Human Enamel." Operative Dentistry 29 (2): 25–30.

Kahler, Bill. 2022. "Present Status and Future Directions – Managing Discoloured Teeth." *International Endodontic Journal* 55 (Suppl 4): 922–950.

Karimi, Mitra, Ali Moradi and John Chen. 2016. "Orofacial Manifestations of Thalassemia." *International Journal of Dentistry* 2016: 287–293.

Kaur, Amanpreet and Kamala Raghavendra. 2021. "Systemic and Developmental Causes of Tooth Discoloration." *Dental Clinics of North America* 65 (1): 112–118.

Kim, Jane W. and James P. Simmer. 2017. "Hereditary Dentin Defects: Molecular Genetics and Clinical Expression." *Journal of Dental Research* 96 (11): 118–126.

Kiran, S. and Harish Prasad. 2017. "Chromogenic Microorganisms in Dental Staining: Clinical Presentation and Management." *Journal of Clinical Pediatric Dentistry* 41 (2): 152–155.

Kugel, G., P. Papathanasiou, M. Ghalili, and P. Perry. 2000. "Clinical Evaluation of a 35% Hydrogen Peroxide In-Office Whitening System." Compendium of Continuing Education in Dentistry 21: 59–66.

Kugel, Gerard, and Sarah Ferreira. 2005. "The Art and Science of Tooth Whitening." Journal of the Massachusetts Dental Society 54 (2): 34–37.

Kwon, S. R., and P. Wertz. 2015. "Review of Bleaching Agents." *Journal of Esthetic and Restorative Dentistry* 27 (5): 12–24.
https://doi.org/10.1111/jerd.12152

Kwon, S. R., and P. Wertz. 2015. "Review of the Mechanism of Tooth Whitening." *Journal of Esthetic and Restorative Dentistry* 27 (5): 13–25.
https://doi.org/10.1111/jerd.12152

Kwon, S. R., O. Kurti, and U. Oyoyo. 2015. "Efficacy of In-Office Tooth Whitening with and without Light Activation." Journal of Dentistry 43 (2): 98–104. https://doi.org/10.1016/j.jdent.2014.06.004

Kwon, Sam and Phillip Wertz. 2015. "Review of Tooth Discoloration and Whitening Agents." *Journal of the American Dental Association* 146 (11 Suppl): S53–S57.

Kwon, Seok-Ho, and Paula Wertz. 2015. "Review of Whitening Agents and Tooth Whitening Techniques." *Journal of Esthetic and Restorative Dentistry* 27 (1): 29–40.

Kwon, So Ran, and Philip W. Wertz. 2015. "Review of the Mechanism of Tooth Whitening." *Journal of Esthetic and Restorative Dentistry* 27 (5): 240–57. https://doi.org/10.1111/jerd.12152.

Laguerre, Amélie, Arnaud Nzihou and Stéphane Viennot. 2021. "Management Strategies for Developmental Tooth Discoloration." *Journal of Esthetic and Restorative Dentistry* 33 (1): 112–119.

Leonard, R. H., et al. 1998. "Nightguard Vital Bleaching: 10% vs 16% Carbamide Peroxide." *Journal of Esthetic Dentistry* 10 (6): 345–354.

Li, Yiming. 1996. "Tooth Bleaching Using Peroxide-Containing Agents." Compendium of Continuing Education in Dentistry 17 (7): 24–31.

Maran, B. M., et al. 2020. "In-office vs. At-home Bleaching: A Systematic Review and Meta-analysis." *Operative Dentistry* 45 (3): 221–233. https://doi.org/10.2341/19-091-L

Maran, B. M., et al. 2020. "Meta-analysis of Bleaching Concentrations." *Operative Dentistry* 45 (3): 221–233. https://doi.org/10.2341/19-091-L

Markowitz, Kenneth. 2010. "An Overview of Tooth Sensitivity." Dental Clinics of North America 54 (1): 61–67. https://doi.org/10.1016/j.cden.2009.08.001

Matis, B. A., et al. 2000. "Clinical Evaluation of Carbamide Peroxide." *Journal of the American Dental Association* 131 (3): 371–379.

Matis, B. A., J. K. Wang, M. A. Cochran, and G. J. Eckert. 2010. "In Vivo Dehydration and Colour Change in Teeth." Journal of Dentistry 38: 129–134. https://doi.org/10.1016/j.jdent.2010.02.001

Matis, B. A., M. A. Cochran, and G. J. Eckert. 2009. "Review of Carbamide Peroxide Whitening Agents." Journal of the American Dental Association 140 (9): 1079–1085. https://doi.org/10.14219/jada.archive.2009.0339

Matis, Bruce A. 2003. "Tray Whitening: What the Evidence Shows." Compendium of Continuing Education in Dentistry 24 (4): 92–101.

Matis, Bruce A. 2016. "Tray Whitening: What the Evidence Shows." *Compendium of Continuing Education in Dentistry* 37 (2): 110–117.

Mena-Serrano, A. P., et al. 2016. “Light-activated vs. Chemically Activated Whitening: Randomized Trial.” *Journal of Dentistry* 50: 56–63. https://doi.org/10.1016/j.jdent.2016.04.006

Mittal, S., et al. 2015. “Comparison of Non-vital Bleaching Agents.” *Journal of Conservative Dentistry* 18 (2): 162–168. https://doi.org/10.4103/0972-0707.153067

Nathoo, S., et al. 2003. “Daily Use Whitening: Clinical Evaluation.” *Journal of Clinical Dentistry* 14 (2): 23–28.

Pallarés-Serrano, A., S. Pallarés-Serrano, A. Pallarés-Serrano, G. Martinez-Martinez, and A. Pallarés-Sabater. 2024. “Comparative Study of the Expansive Behaviour of Different Internal Bleaching Agents.” *Applied Sciences* 14 (2): 532. https://doi.org/10.3390/app14020532

Patil, Gauri, Amit Reche and Priyanka Paul. 2022. “Tooth Bleaching and Its Adverse Effects: A Review.” *Journal of Pharmaceutical Research International* 34 (57): 35–44.

Pindobilowo, Pindobilowo, Dwi Ariani and Fauziah M. Asim. 2024. “Effects of Dental Bleaching Treatment Ingredients and Their Influence on the Hardness of Tooth Enamel.” *Formosa Journal of Applied Sciences* 3 (3): 987–1002.

Plotino, G., A. Buono, and N. M. Grande. 2019. “Non-Vital Tooth Bleaching: A Review of Materials, Indications, and Techniques.” International Endodontic Journal 52 (5): 740–752.

Plotino, Gianluca, and Nicola M. Grande. 2019. “Management of Tooth Discoloration.” *Endodontic Topics* 38 (1): 111–125. DOI: https://doi.org/10.1111/etp.12220

Potocnik, I., D. Kosec, and D. Gaspersic. 2005. “Effect of 10% Carbamide Peroxide on Enamel Microhardness.” Journal of Endodontics 26 (2): 95–98. https://doi.org/10.1016/S0099-2399(00)80218-1

Ranganath, Lakshmi R., John C. Jarvis and Josie A. Gallagher. 2019. “Ochronosis and Alkaptonuria: Clinical and Molecular Insights.” *QJM: An International Journal of Medicine* 112 (12): 855–863.

Rotstein, I., M. Friedman, and Z. Torek. 1993. “Effect of Different Bleaching Techniques on Tooth Colour and Microhardness.” Journal of Endodontics 19 (6): 266–269.

Rotstein, I., Z. Torek, and M. Friedman. 1991. "Bleaching of Discoloured Non-Vital Teeth: Sodium Perborate with Distilled Water vs. 30% Hydrogen Peroxide." Journal of Endodontics 17 (5): 845–849.

Santos, Juliana, and Gustavo Souza. 2018. "Tooth Discoloration Induced by Endodontic Sealers: A Critical Review." *Restorative Dentistry & Endodontics* 43 (4): 231–239. DOI: https://doi.org/10.5395/rde.2018.43.e49

Siddiqui, Sana, and Arif Khan. 2016. "Metallic Ion Migration and Amalgam-Induced Discoloration: An Updated Review." *Journal of Conservative Dentistry* 19 (1): 85–92. DOI: https://doi.org/10.4103/0972-0707.173199

Silva, L. F., R. Carvalho, and T. Azevedo. 2021. "Safety and Effectiveness of Intracoronal Bleaching Agents: A Systematic Review." Materials 14 (3): 1–12.

Silva, Mayra J., George W. Suckling and Eleanor Vierrou. 2020. "Enamel Hypoplasia: Etiology, Diagnosis and Management." *International Journal of Paediatric Dentistry* 30 (1): 33–39.

Sulieman, M. 2004. "An Overview of Tooth-Whitening Techniques." British Dental Journal 196 (7): 414–423. https://doi.org/10.1038/sj.bdj.4811074

Sulieman, M. 2005. "An Overview of Tooth Discolouration: Extrinsic, Intrinsic and Internalized Stains." *Dental Update* 32 (8): 463–471. https://doi.org/10.12968/denu.2005.32.8.463

Sulieman, M., et al. 2004. "Hydrogen Peroxide Whitening Systems: Efficacy and Mechanisms." *Dental Update* 31 (7): 401–408.

Sundell, Anna L. and Goran Koch. 2020. "Developmental Defects of Enamel and Dentin." *European Archives of Paediatric Dentistry* 21 (2): 85–93.

Tay, L. Y., M. R. Koseoglu, S. L. Carvalho, J. A. Duarte, and S. L. S. Afonso. 2009. "Effect of Home Bleaching Agents on Resin Composite Surface Roughness." Brazilian Dental Journal 20 (2): 101–105. https://doi.org/10.1590/S0103-64402009000200006

Thosre, Deepak, and Shilpa Mulay. 2009. "Smile Enhancement the Conservative Way: Tooth Whitening Procedures." *Journal of Conservative Dentistry* 12 (4): 164–168. https://doi.org/10.4103/0972-0707.58342

Torabinejad, Mahmoud, Ahmad Abdel-Fouad and Richard Walton. 2022. *Endodontics: Principles and Practice,* 6th ed. St. Louis: Elsevier. Pages 213–219.

Valles, Maria, and Alexandra Mercade. 2015. "Coronal Tooth Discoloration Related to Bismuth Oxide in MTA." *Journal of Endodontics* 41 (2): 255–259.
DOI: https://doi.org/10.1016/j.joen.2014.10.009

Vazquez, Lorenzo and Marcel Wagner. 2016. "Metal-Induced Tooth Discolouration: Clinical Characteristics and Management." *International Dental Journal* 66 (4): 287–290.

Vilhena, F. V., et al. 2019. "Efficacy and Safety of Carbamide Peroxide." *Clinical Oral Investigations* 23 (1): 215–224.
https://doi.org/10.1007/s00784-018-2422-3

Vilhena, F. V., et al. 2019. "Efficacy of High-concentration Hydrogen Peroxide: A Clinical Trial." *Clinical Oral Investigations* 23 (1): 215–224.
https://doi.org/10.1007/s00784-018-2422-3

Watts, Andrew and Martin Addy. 2019. "Intrinsic Tooth Discoloration: A Review of Aetiology and Management." *British Dental Journal* 226 (11): 151–159.

Weiger, R., S. Kuhn, and A. Löst. 1994. "Effect of Sodium Perborate on Colour of Non-Vital Teeth." Journal of Endodontics 20 (2): 93–95.

Wright, Jonathan T., Katherine Carrion and Sydney Hill. 2015. "Amelogenesis Imperfecta: Updated Review of Clinical Features and Genetics." *Pediatric Dentistry* 37 (2): 143–151.

Yu, Bin, Jin-Soo Ahn, and Yong-Keun Lee. 2009. "Measurement of Translucency of Tooth Enamel and Dentin." *Acta Odontologica Scandinavica* 67 (6): 367-372.
https://doi.org/10.1080/00016350802577818

Yu, H., L. Li, Y. Cheng, Z. Han, and X. Zhao. 2011. "Effects of Whitening Strips on Tooth Colour and Enamel Structure." Journal of Dentistry 39 (3): 43–48. https://doi.org/10.1016/j.jdent.2011.01.002

Zijp, J. R., H. van der Meulen, and J. W. van der Meulen. 2016. "Measurements and Modelling of the Influence of Dentine Colour and Enamel on Tooth Colour." *Journal of Dentistry* 43 (3): 327-333.
https://doi.org/10.1016/j.jdent.2014.01.006